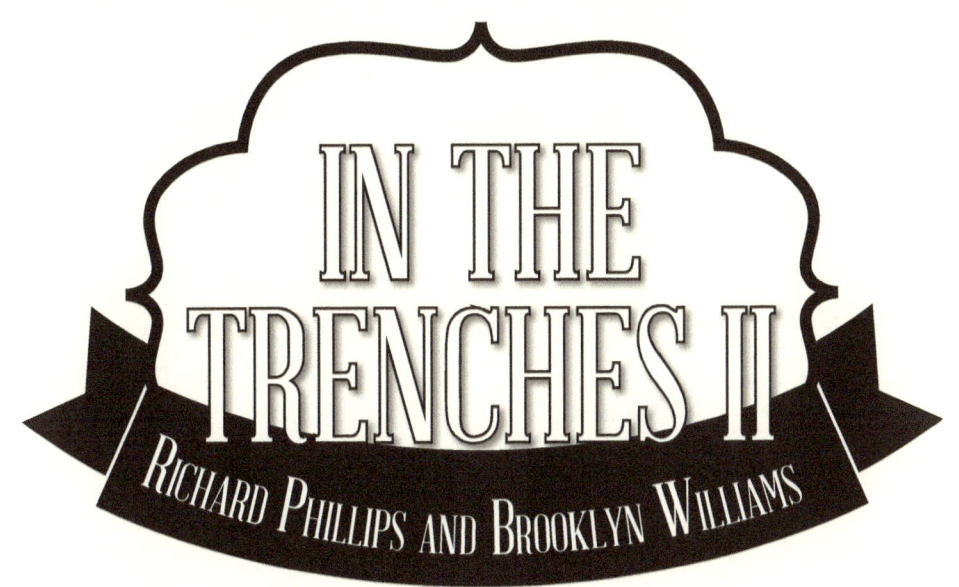

IN THE TRENCHES II

RICHARD PHILLIPS AND BROOKLYN WILLIAMS

authorHOUSE®

AuthorHouse™
1663 Liberty Drive
Bloomington, IN 47403
www.authorhouse.com
Phone: 1 (800) 839-8640

Published by AuthorHouse   06/22/2016

ISBN: 978-1-4969-6540-0 (sc)
ISBN: 978-1-4969-6539-4 (hc)
ISBN: 978-1-4969-6538-7 (e)

Library of Congress Control Number: 2015900960

Print information available on the last page.

Any people depicted in stock imagery provided by Thinkstock are models, and such images are being used for illustrative purposes only. Certain stock imagery © Thinkstock.

This book is printed on acid-free paper.

By telling my story, it is hoped that this book will tell people about my war, and help people who are fighting obesity, glucose control, High Blood Pressure or, perhaps something else. This may help them understand that they are not alone, and that <u>there is hope</u>, that tomorrow can be new day, and that victory, in many cases, is there for the taking.

If there is a central theme to this story, it is hope!

In The Trenches II

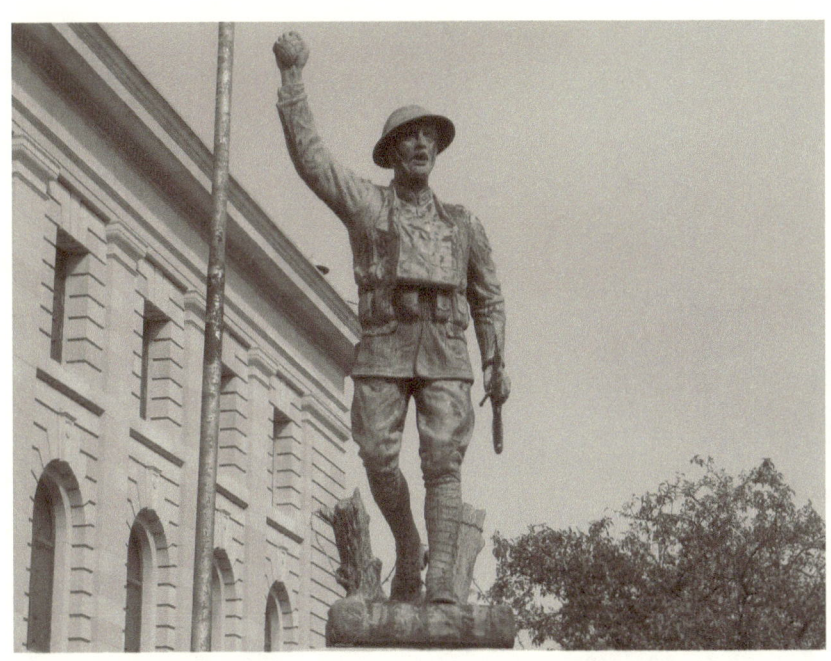

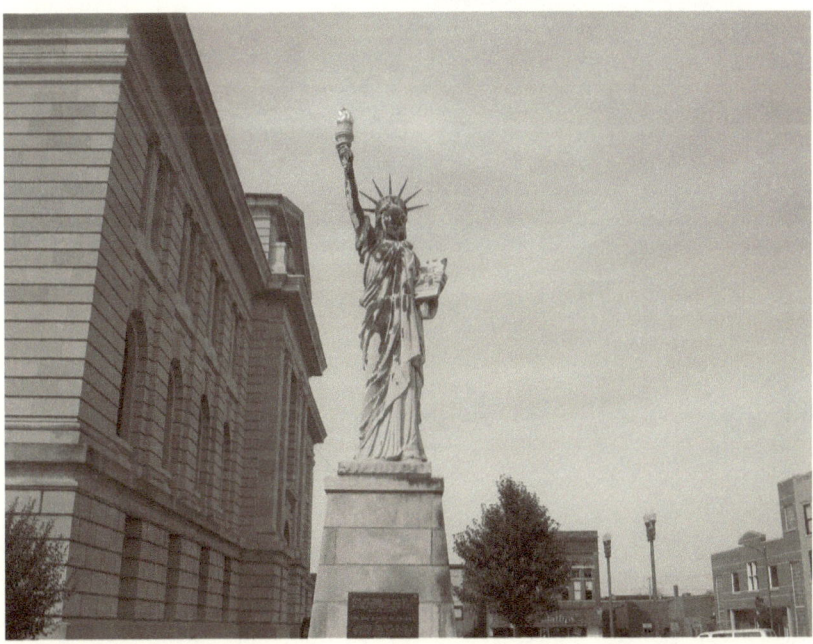

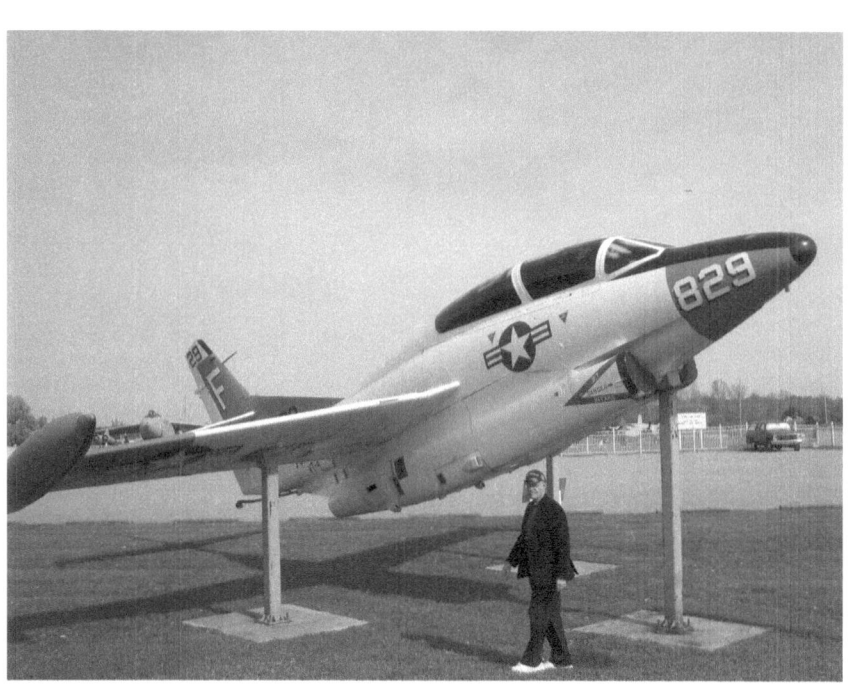

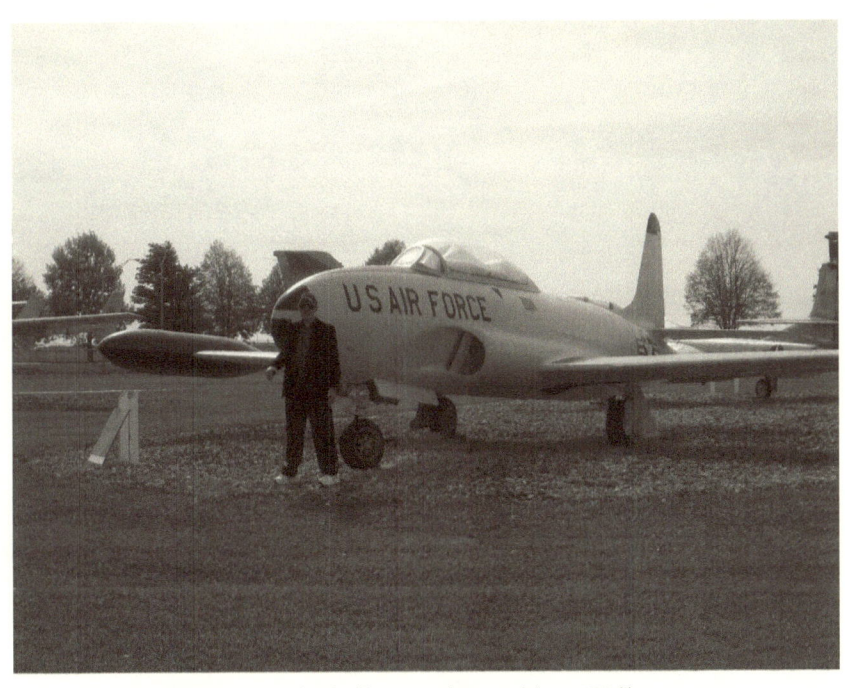

By: Richard Phillips and Brooklyn Williams
10/2/14

In The Trenches II

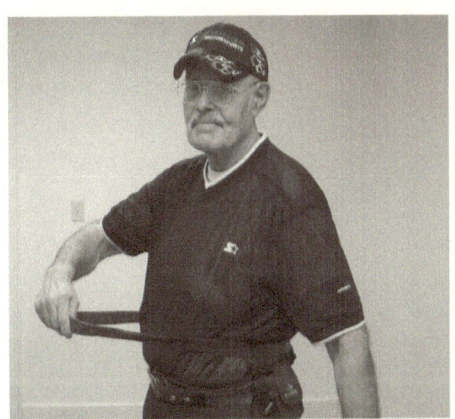 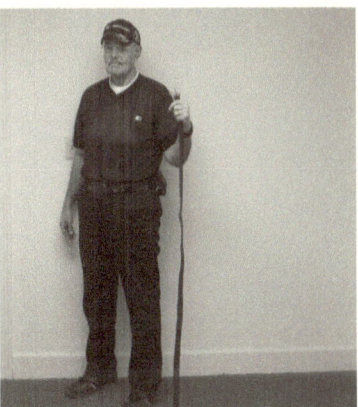

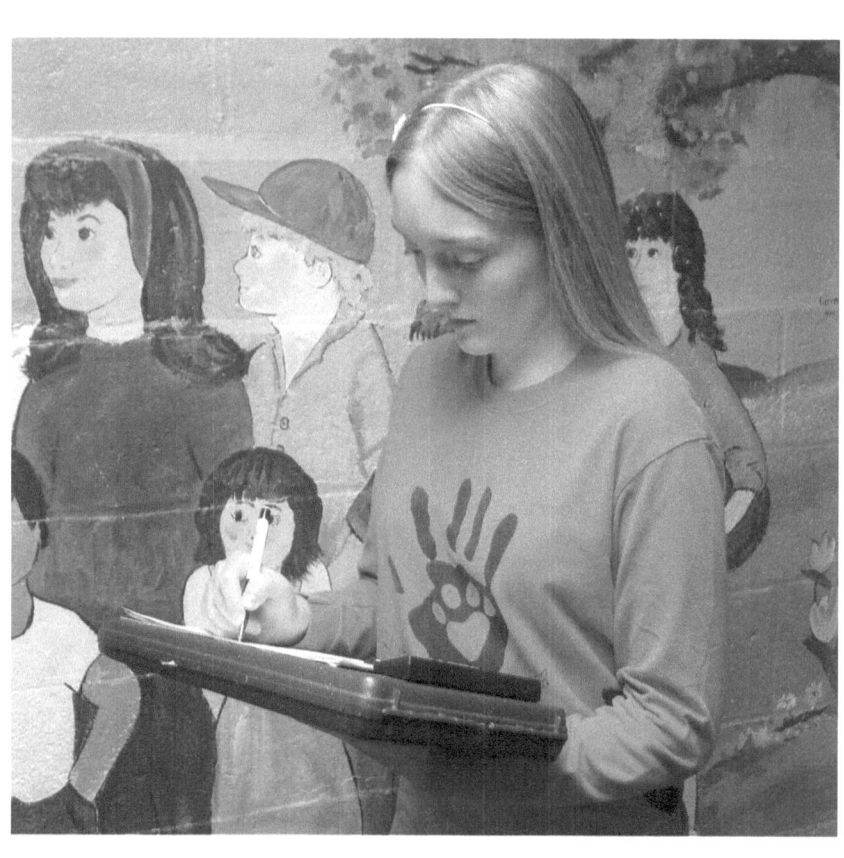

We want to take this opportunity to thank the many people who have encouraged us along the way. The power of people is simply amazing, and we are in their debt. During the early part of this journey, the encouragement played a large role in staying the course and building resolve. The temptation to go back to old habits was very strong. Our thanks go to these people, some of whom are recent advocates.

Blessings to all of you!

Gary Colby
Randy Cress
Kent Cress
Karen Shidler
Ron & Mary Ann Scher
Dean & Patsy Spear
Jaime Kinsey
Nina Lynch
Will & Nancy and Warren Pennie
Albert Leazenby
Dan and Mindy Gehle

Contents

About the Authors

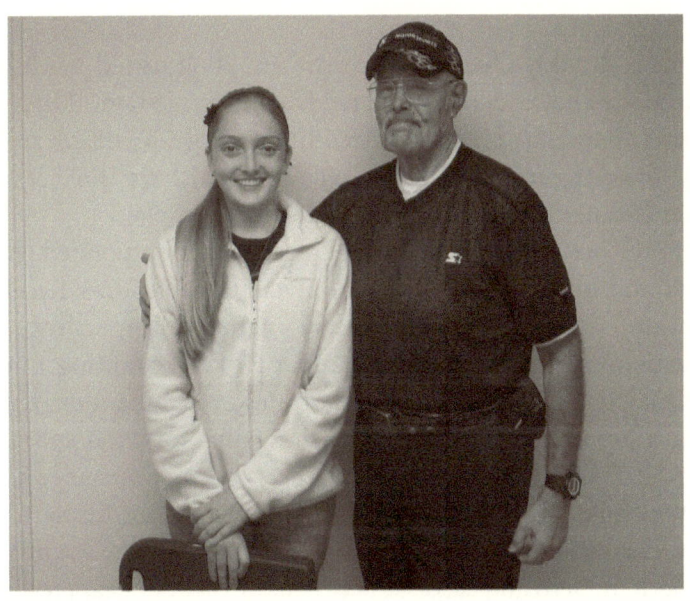

I am Richard Phillips, Born in Watsonville California, raised in California in both the Redwoods and the coastal areas of San Francisco to Monterey, California. I graduated from Santa Cruz High School, Santa Cruz California, went into the Army in 1961 and was honorably discharged in 1964. I went to College at Cabrillo College and majored in Electronics. I went to Hartnell College and majored in Business Administration and graduated in 1969. I attended Monterey Peninsula College and studied Computer programming. I also took course studies at Purdue University-environmental studies/Hazardous Materials Policy and Application, Indiana University/Indianapolis-Business Law and the University of Cincinnati-project management.

My background is manufacturing with specialization in Industrial Engineering/MTM, Statistical Process Control, Production Control, Safety, Management, Management Information Systems, and Supervision. I was also responsible for Training/SPC-Management-Supervision,.

My hobbies include basketball, woodworking, gardening, fishing, music/ guitar, songwriting, and photography. I also operate a close tolerance machining business.

I enjoy writing, spending time with my grandchildren, and I participate in community service through two local churches and our Local Mexico Indiana Lions Club.

My name is Brooklyn Sierra Williams, I am 20 years old. I was born in Peru, Indiana and recently graduated from North Miami High School in Denver, Indiana. I will be attending college in the near future, possibly majoring in a field involving animals. I have three cats of my own and I sometimes fill in at our local animal shelter.

I am the Office manager at R & L Phillips, Incorporated, Mexico, Indiana, and am responsible for all invoicing, Accounts Receivables, production accounting, computer maintenance, filing, office organization, wireless computer backup, EFTPS accounting, Customer data management, Standard operating Procedure maintenance, PDF File Creation and storage, EFT transfers, directory and subdirectory creation and maintenance, Outlook Express File maintenance and I am also responsible for the appearance of all our standard forms.

My interests include playing the guitar; I really enjoy the country music genre, both modern and classic. I occasionally make appearances playing my guitar at our local churches. It's something I very much enjoy. Taylor Swift is my idol. She has been one of my biggest inspirations for wanting to learn guitar from the beginning. I also participate in community services by helping our local Mexico Indiana Lions Club at dinners and breakfasts.

Some other interests of mine include writing poetry, playing basketball, watching movies, and crocheting.

Introduction

In The Trenches

In The Trenches is a story of a war. This is a personal war. It is a clear description of many battles and the fact that I lost most of those battles in the beginning. That period of losing the war lasted for decades and there were numerous failures, before reaching some success.

The war, at least at first, was against obesity. As that war raged on for several years, two other major fights took place. As I was fighting battles against obesity, and losing, diabetes entered the picture. Then, before winning either the war against excessive weight or diabetes, another fight emerged. I developed High Blood Pressure.

The fight against diabetes lasted for years. It was that battle that brought things to a head and actually put me in a state of desperation. It was this battle, diabetes, which led to the writing of this book. Glucose was the first thing that was documented in this book.

This story is going to attempt to bring understanding about what caused my failures and what was done to reach success. It is also going to reveal that I did not have a real measure of success, until after I reached a point of desperation and reached out to GOD. This story is going to expose a change from the first few sentences you just read. Notice the I's.

Throughout the period of failures, there were 3 things that became evident:

The first thing was the emphasis on I. I decided. I did. I suffered the consequences. In short, I relied upon my own wisdom, which was, and is, very limited, to choose how I would deal with my battle, rather than rely upon the guidance of those who were seasoned veterans on the war against obesity. I wanted to have my cake and eat it too. Seems appropriate, doesn't it!

The second thing that became obvious, after a lot of time passed, was that I did NOT understand. Had I understood, maybe I would have listened.

Finally, the last thing being that I did NOT listen.

If you are at a place in your life where you have reached a point of desperation, this process may be for you.

How can you be miserable and not know it? That will also be explained.

There is going to be an emphasis on certain fundamentals that are crucial to my continuing success. These fundamentals are:

Prayer
Humbleness
Building resolve
Identifying balance
Keep the doctor informed
Understanding advertisements
Anticipation
Getting out what you put in
Smiling and laughter
Stress
Time investment
Doubt
Awareness
Taking charge

Exercise
Feedback
Understanding
Results
Motivation
Success
Patience
Staying the course
Cause and effect
Desperation
Self control
Cost vs. Benefit
Panning for GOLD
Listening
System overload
Breaking The Routine-The Planned Reward

We will talk about "The Daily Routine", which embraces the new direction of my life. It covers a (9) nine year period that began on July 15th, 2005 and continues to this day. A lot of the references or topics are entered at different times, during this (9) nine year period.

The variety of headings helps to reinforce concepts and fundamentals which are vital to this process.

By telling my story, it is hoped that this book will tell people about my war, and help people who are fighting obesity, glucose control, High Blood Pressure or, perhaps something else. This may help them understand that they are not alone, and that there is Hope, that tomorrow can be new day, and that victory, in many cases, is there for the taking.

If there is a central theme to this story, it is Hope!

My Story

I am not a Medical Professional.

My name is Richard Phillips. This is my story. I was obese for many years. After losing a substantial amount of weight, and keeping it off, many acquaintances and friends suggested that I write a book. This is a novel, pardon the pun, approach to weight management, and does not promote a specific diet. *It is a process, not a diet*. I refer to it as "The Daily Routine" &/or"*Eating For Effect*."

"The Daily Routine", which plays a large role in managing my weight, glucose, and blood pressure, will be described, soon. But, before I address that process, I want to provide some background information.

History

In the Trenches is a story of many failures, before success. It is a story about a personal war with myself. It is a story about a person who fought obesity for about 25 years (and lost most of the time) and then diabetes, type 2 for about (7) years, before discovering something that would have a life changing effect. I call it answered prayer.

Years ago, in the seventies, weight began to accumulate. I had weighed about 185 pounds in 1973. I was 31 and had become a manufacturing supervisor, specializing in manufacturing administration and industrial engineering-(MTM). I had been at 185 pounds for several years, with minor fluctuations. This was my normal weight. As I rose through the ranks of management, I spent more time planning, and less time directing. Consequently, my physical activity on the job lessened. I decided to supplement my lack of activity with a weekly regimen at the local YMCA, three times a week. This went on for a few years.

As I continued to rise in management, to the position of 'Plant Manager', my responsibilities increased. As a result, I spent more time on the job. I became less physically active, and finally scheduled no time for the YMCA. In my forties, I began to get too heavy, and would go through the process of fighting weight control with radical steps, trying to overcome the excess weight. These were not recommended steps, but were things that I did to lose weight that were absolutely wrong. I had limited success, but was not really addressing the true problem. The real problem remained masked for years.

Metabolism

Some of the radical steps included skipping meals. This happened before I was discovered with type 2 diabetes. After I was diagnosed with type 2 diabetes and after I took medication for diabetes, sometimes, I would eat only once a day, in order to get my glucose levels to a safe value. If that didn't work I would skip a day and then decide to eat. If that still did not work, I would skip two days. At the very end of this process, I actually skipped a total of 4 days. At that time, we were looking at the year 2005. I was battling type 2 diabetes as well as obesity, and losing most of the battles.

It is my belief, even though I am not a medical professional, that metabolism is the process the body uses to convert food into energy. Energy equals glucose. The body appears to have a wonderful management system to control a variety of very complex activities. Endocrine glands play a major role in this activity. When we, as human beings, fail to listen to medical professionals who almost always say "eat several small meals a day", we can create a nightmare for ourselves. That is exactly what I did. When we make sudden changes in behavior, such as skipping meals, there appears to be a reaction to those specific changes. It is definitely not favorable. I was guilty of making bad decisions, thinking I was going to achieve my goals, without realizing I was creating the foundation for significant trouble.

After reducing the frequency of eating by skipping meals, in some cases for days and days, the body just seemed to conserve fat at a much higher level and/or degree, and just did not convert food into energy very quickly. Things just seemed to slow down. The end result was, I simply did not lose much weight and other things may have stopped occurring that should have been happening in order to metabolize food adequately.

If you love food and have found yourself rationalizing and thinking about trying to find a way to avoid eating several small meals a day, think about the dilemma that I created.

Yet, there is <u>Hope</u>!

Diabetes Discovered

Let's go back in time, just a bit.

In 1995, I weighed over three hundred pounds. The analog scales, which were not too accurate, actually showed I weighed 344 pounds. I was so large that I could not be seated at a restaurant that had fixed chairs-to-table arrangements. It was also a tight arrangement for the steering wheel in my car and my stomach. I finally began to take more drastic steps to curb the weight problem and did drop to about 275 pounds. Remember, this was the first war. It was <u>the war against obesity</u>, which had lasted for decades. Those drastic steps included skipping meals.

Three years later, it was 1998. It was then that I was diagnosed with type 2 diabetes. This was an accidental discovery through an insurance examination. My glucose was reported at over 580. My doctor was emphatic about dieting, losing weight, and exercising. He was a good man. A couple of hours prior to the blood test, I had eaten a huge breakfast with sausage, eggs, and pancakes. I knew that probably caused the numbers to be high. I asked him to give me two additional weeks to diet and exercise to see if that would make a difference. He agreed. I took the time, and then took another test. The numbers were lower, but I was still diagnosed with type 2 diabetes. As I grappled with this problem, there were several things I really needed to know. How would I react to medication? Would I have to take medication forever? What effects would diabetes have upon me and what could I do about it? *What was diabetes?*
Why did I become a person with diabetes? Could this problem be reversed?

This is one of those things in life that I would describe as a major change. My life would not be the same, and there was a certain amount of apprehension. A lot of that was caused by not anticipating the fact that

I would become a person with diabetes and not know a thing about diabetes.

Even though this was such an undesired event, it may have been something that ultimately resulted in a positive outcome. This may sound strange, and I did not know it at the time, but, suddenly having diabetes could have been a blessing!

<u>Research</u>

One of the good things that I did was take training in nutrition and diabetes at a local hospital. There was training for several hours over a two week period in each discipline. This was very helpful. Yet, there was a tremendous amount of information that I needed to know in order to get a real understanding of both nutrition and diabetes. I did a lot of research. When I researched diabetes, I would look for definitions and for terms that I did not understand. There were many. Research led me to various new words that I had never heard of or had not previously known. I checked computer encyclopedias like Wikipedia, and searched to understand diabetes. I began to form opinions about such items as Neural Transmitters, the Hypothalamus, the Pancreas, Polypeptide Hormones, and other terms, and the relationships between these components.

After collecting some information, I made some good decisions, but I also made some <u>very bad decisions</u>. *Here was a really bad one*! For years, prior to being discovered with type 2 diabetes, I had skipped meals, and then, when I did eat, I over-ate. The truth is, eating became an obsessive pleasure. Once I had routinely eaten for pleasure, I looked forward to the experience and actually over ate almost every day! In retrospect, that was an abuse of my system. There were numerous bad effects from years of skipping meals. Yet, at the time, I had no idea what I was doing. I did not know that what I did could cause so many problems. Did skipping meals cause diabetes? It probably did.
Did obesity cause diabetes? It probably did. Did eating giant meals cause diabetes? It probably did. If there was something that people did or could do to cause diabetes, I probably did it. Do I know for certain that these things caused diabetes? No.

As I said before, most medical professionals had stressed moderation, eating frequently, and eating small meals. This advice was not something new, however, <u>I did it my way.</u> That was the wrong way. <u>I did not listen</u>. Furthermore, even though I heard their words, <u>I absolutely did not understand</u> the consequences of doing it my way.

It is one thing to hear something, and quite another to understand it. With me, understanding usually occurs when the "why" is part of the explanation. If I understand the mechanics of what happens, I have a better chance to understand it. If I understand it, there is a better chance that logic will prevail. There is no question that I did not understand the "Why" or the "How" when it came to eating small meals several times a day.
That is not an excuse, but it is a simple or complex fact, depending on one's point of view.

After researching diabetes, a mental picture began to form, and I took certain steps, which did bring my glucose under control. The real problem was, I failed to listen to the professionals and attempted to handle this my own way. I rationalized that if I ate once a day, I could still enjoy many of the foods that I enjoyed at the quantity to which I was accustomed. I said this earlier and repeated it again and will likely keep repeating it. Why? I am sure the reader has a brain and can retain information, but the fact is, I had a war going on and I was losing. Why? The opponent was very powerful. More of the why will be explained later, but just understand this. Part of my obesity was caused simply by loving food, eating food, enjoying food, and focusing on food. But, there is more to it.

So, if I repeat the idea about eating giant sized meals, most of which were the last meal of the day, it is because of a near addiction to the powerful sensations that go along with eating the wrong foods. Bear with me. If you are fighting obesity, my guess is that you will have been fighting the same battles I did, and, you will have suffered losses just like me.

There is <u>Hope</u>.

System Overload

The fact is, I could consume about the same amount of food or more at one time as I would if I had eaten several times a day. At least, that was my (incorrect) thinking. With that line of thinking, there was no thought of how much unnecessary stress that I would place upon my body by eating that much food at one time. In my defense, there was little explanation about <u>overloading the system.</u> What I mean by that is simple. By eating way too much at one time, in order to handle higher levels of glucose, I would have to produce more insulin than I would if I had only eaten a small amount of food. The end result is what I call "System Overload".

The doctors were and are right about eating small amounts of food several times a day. That is absolutely good advice and there are several reasons for why that works. At that time, however, there was little explanation about why. Why should I eat small meals and why should I eat several times a day and why should I eat at the same times of day? I do not know if that has changed (giving the explanation of why), but the fact is, eating large meals creates "<u>System Overload</u>". The more food I eat, the more glucose that is created and the more insulin and other polypeptide hormones that are required to keep the system in balance. That is the main selling point regarding eating small meals. Small meals require less support and large meals require more support. That boils down to the fact that the body is going to have to work harder in order to provide balance for large meals. There are other factors that will be discussed such as predictable eating habits and system programming that all help achieve system balance. None the less, I probably would have done it my way anyway. Remember, a lot of this is what I think. For example, I think that our systems, glucose, weight, blood pressure, and others, follow an internal program. The body expects to create so many hormones to perform so many functions, under certain conditions. When we abuse our systems, we likely help change the programs to our disadvantage. This may not be right, but it is the way that I look at it.

We have to remember the term balance, which is discussed later in this book.

From 1998 through the end of 2002, I maintained reasonably good glucose control, but I remained too heavy and I developed some problems with high blood pressure. Over time, the control of glucose became worse, medicine was added, and finally 2005 arrived, with significant problems.

Although I stepped up the exercise (another good decision), and reduced my intake, (also another good choice), it was not enough. I had to take more oral medication, including more dieting and exercise. For a while, that worked, but, over a 3 year period (2002-2005), control was lost. Even though I had dropped to about 260 pounds, I still weighed way too much and had trouble controlling my glucose.

Since a normal weight for me had been, in the distant past, 185 pounds, two hundred and sixty pounds was still terribly over weight. It was easy to look at it from the point of view that I had lost about 84 pounds. That resulted in a mental position of saying, good for me. That's great! I failed to really understand I needed to reach a normal weight level. I also did not realize what the extra 75 pounds was doing to me, my knees and hip joints, and my system.

I did not understand, yet, there was Hope.

The Trip

In 2005, something happened. My wife and I took a trip across the US that resulted in a dramatic and potentially permanent change in our lives. In fact, several changes were made as a result of that trip.

As we traveled, by car (from Indiana to Oregon), across our great land, I had time to reflect upon many issues. One of the things I re- discovered is we have a big and beautiful country. I discovered something else. When I was home, I was so busy, that I had not taken time to face obesity squarely in the face. I had not really gotten on my knees and asked _GOD_ for help. I didn't take the time to address a lot of things that needed attention. I had forgotten how beautiful America was, because I was too busy with work or too busy doing benevolent things, such as serving the local church, the local Lions Club, the United Way, the Cub Scouts, the Local JayCees, the Chamber of Commerce, &/or the

Mexico Community Fact Finding Committee activity. Several local residents volunteered numerous hours to help unravel a long standing problem relating to the discharge of raw sewage into the Eel River, in Mexico, Indiana. The MCFFC was a two year project by itself, and I was the chairman.

The Walls Of Familiarity

The trip that I had just completed exemplified, to the nth degree, an explanation I had given a student going for her thesis who asked why people go to festivals. It was at a breakfast in Rockville, Indiana, with several other people present. I did go to festivals often, so I was a logical person to ask. At least, I did in those days. I thought about her question and then realized that it wasn't the festival that was most important, it was the trip from one place to another that was significant. I was able to see new things, and sometimes different things. It was what happened during the trip to the festival that mattered as much, and maybe more, than the festival itself.

Before taking these small trips, my observations of my immediate surroundings seemed to fade over time. I referred to this phenomenon, the lack of observation, as "The Walls Of Familiarity."

If that is true, how does this relate to "The Daily Routine"? For me, the process of taking a small trip, even though it might not last very long, was a stress reliever. When I returned home, I simply felt better. I not only saw things that were right in front of me that I had not noticed before the trip, but it was as if I had my batteries recharged. This is very likely a natural effect that many people can experience.

If a small trip is a stress reliever, it very likely could have positive effects on glucose levels. As for weight management, it probably had the reverse effect, because I usually have a tendency to eat the wrong things on trips, though since 2005, that has changed too. Now, it is much easier to stay on the path set out in "The Daily Routine."

In 2005, the trip that was taken was a little different. In that case, even though the "Walls of Familiarity" really collapsed, the destination revealed wonderful young relatives who were thrilled to meet us, and/or who were likely responsible for adding so much to our lives. You could just see their love in their eyes as they excitedly shared their lives with us. Though we did not get to stay long, there was something very special and powerful that we experienced.

The bottom line here is this. If you get a chance to get away for short periods of time, there are possible benefits from this that may actually help on your journey in life.

The Change

When we returned from our trip, we were not the same. Something was added to us on that trip. I knew it and I did ask _GOD_ to preserve it. I cannot fully describe the sensation, other than to say that we seemed to be much more complete.

Upon returning, we made a few changes immediately. We sat down and put together a 22 page letter, which described our recent journey. We burned cds, which included 570 high resolution photos of family and friends and sent 22 families copies. We then identified some of the things that we needed to do and met with some of our friends in Indiana. We decided to take the summer off from most benevolent activities and focus on things that needed to be done. We amassed a list of over 100 items and put it in writing. We completed over 70 tasks, during the summer. We continued to support our local Lions Club and our church, but we did budget our time.

Stress

When we worry we create stress. According to the medical profession, stress is an element that causes glucose levels to rise. I have proof of that. There are a lot of words that describe stress. Here are a few: pressure, strain, anxiety, tension, trauma, hassle, urgency, emphasis, disturbance, shock, or upset. It's my belief that stress causes a lot of trouble for the human body.

It's a known fact that stress elevates glucose levels. Later in the book, we will describe a specific event that caused my glucose to be elevated. When we think about pressure, or strain or shock, we think about things that happen to most people. It has often been said that it's not what happens to us that makes the difference, but how we react to what happens to us. In spite of how we think or react, stress still manages to take its toll.

Stress, for success to happen under this system, needs to be managed. Not taking time for ourselves can create a lot of stress. Not determining what is important in our life can also lead to stress. This relates back to balance. One of the things that helps identify stress and provide understanding relates to collecting information on events that are stress related. Here are a few things that may cause stress: events such as: public speaking, public disputes, private disputes, being late for appointments, family matters, public performances, or anything that might cause us to worry and lead to anxiety. Someone we care about who goes to the hospital, contracts cancer, has a fire, has a car accident, looses a job, (or has some other traumatic event) can lead to stress. It does not have to happen directly to us to be stressful. Many times, these are things that are out of our control, yet they may be troublesome. When that happens, you can almost be certain that stress will be involved. Being aware of this can at least give you a heads up and help you decide if you need to do anything special to help manage stress.

Out Of Balance

So, following the trip, we took the summer off from most benevolent activities and budgeted our time. These things, (the numerous benevolent things), were all good things, and I have no regret for being involved in those activities. I simply did not establish a balance. This is part of my nature, when addressing things that need to be done. That is to say that I try to give 100% on a project, and focus tightly on it, while other needs either don't get addressed or don't get the time they deserve. Time to wind down and recharge is often ignored. Today, a different strategy would likely be used. The project would still need to be undertaken. Instead of manning the operation and managing it, I would likely seek an ally or two and delegate authority and responsibility to "Make it

Happen". When looking at balance, I have to recognize that there are only so many hours in a day. How do I want to spend those hours? How can I divide those hours into a routine where an appropriate amount of time is given, to accomplish personal goals? As the Book of Proverbs says "There is a season for all things." Translation, there is a time for all things. Balance to me means giving the right amount of time to each item of importance, at the right time. What were those items of importance? In days gone by, that just wasn't in my thinking. How could I have balance, if I did not realize I was out of balance? How could I have balance if I did not take the time to identify items of importance that needed time? I did not understand. Now, one thing that helps balance my day is to put the items of importance in writing and assign a theoretical time to allot for each major activity. Looking at those items helps awareness and helps me spend the right amount of time on each component. That, putting it in writing, helps me achieve balance. It also helps me to not have too much to do on a given day. If the schedule has too many hours in it, I can simply trim either the number of things to do, or drop the allotted time for some of the functions. Either choice helps keep me in balance.

Time

None the less, a trip, which began on March 27, 2005 and ended on April 17, 2005, gave me *time* that I had not taken previously. *Time to review my life. Time to meet old acquaintances and new ones. Time* to reflect. And, perhaps nearly the most important, *time* to be enveloped with unconditional love from so many wonderful people from Indiana to California to Oregon and Arizona. Finally, the most important thing was to take *time* to pray.

Doctor's Diagnosis

In 2005, I had seen my doctor and had spoken to two of his nurses on different occasions. This was before July 15th, 2005. Remember, we had returned from our trip in April. *The message was loud and clear*. I had to lose weight. I was at the limit of oral medication for diabetes, and, if the newly prescribed medication failed to work, insulin was the next step.

In that case, that meant that I would have to take shots to manage my diabetes. The newly prescribed medicine was in addition to 4 pills that I was already taking to manage diabetes. That meant that when it arrived, I would be taking five pills a day to manage diabetes. Unbelievable!

That is when I put my hands in the air, figuratively speaking, and asked _GOD_ for help. I was in trouble, and I knew it. There is an old saying that goes like this. "When I'm down on my knees is when I'm closest to heaven." I was going to the source. I was beginning to realize that my way was not working. My back was against the wall with a gun to my head. I was beginning to realize that I was in trouble. Perhaps this was the beginning of understanding.

Prayer

I realized that what I had been doing, for years, was not effective, and, it may have been the cause for some, or all, of my medical troubles. It was July 14th, 2005. While continuing to battle obesity, glucose control, and high blood pressure, I did seriously ask _GOD_ for help. I needed to know how to establish weight control and manage my diabetes. I needed to know what to do. The new medication, in addition to older medications for diabetes, would arrive soon. While I waited for it to arrive, I prayed and spoke with friends. The prayer admitted my failure to seek _GOD's_ help. It was a failure to really address obesity as well as my other problems and it was a prayer asking for help. With that prayer, there was Hope!

Answered Prayer

My prayers were answered. _On July 15th, 2005, I took a new direction._ It wasn't easy, but, as time went by, it became routine. I decided to use much of the training I had received in manufacturing respective to process analysis. College training in management was put to use. Planning, Organizing, Directing, Coordinating, and Controlling, the five main elements of management, would be intensely used. Some Statistical Process Control tools were used too. Standard Deviation, Range, and Averages were attached to behavioral charts. These were employed along with trend analysis. I applied these elements to my diabetes, and weight and blood pressure problems.

In addition, I was going to change the food that I was eating and drinking. In discussions with our friends, Frank and Velma Townsend, I decided to start eating things like Zucchini squash from our garden on a frequent basis. Since we had a garden, I also would eat a lot of fresh tomatoes. Red meats were out, breads were a no-no, and potatoes and carbonated drinks were simply banned.
This was a major change!

This was not a diet out of a book. It was a direction I felt the need to follow, the day following my prayer of desperation. I would also try micro waving eggs without butter for breakfast, and would purchase an *accurate digital scale*. I would take *multiple glucose readings,* during the day. Over time, I added all the information, including *blood pressure*, *glucose,* and *weight* readings. These were entered onto a chart. Additionally, I would record items such as solid and liquid intake, stress, coffee, sleep, and exercise and I would run correlations against weight, blood pressure, and glucose levels. I would then analyze the medicine I was taking, the time of day such medicine was taken and check the results. I would also check with my doctor to ensure that these changes were approved and seek his advice. The number of variables, items that I kept track of, grew as the months passed.

Collecting the information, without assuming too much, followed Statistical Process Control methods, and using the same process to find results that I used on the manufacturing floor, when evaluating a particular process turned out to be a big help, when I analyzed glucose, weight and or BP data.

Why do all of this? Just like a manufacturing process that I needed to understand, I wanted to know what was happening. I wanted to learn and understand how my systems were behaving. By learning about my systems, weight, glucose, and blood pressure, and documenting what was happening, I could possibly establish data that might allow me to know what had happened, what was happening and then, possibly help me influence what would happen.

It was a lofty idea that I had looked at in 1998, but this time, there was a powerful element added, as well as some additional fundamentals that would be put into practice.

This was the beginning of "The Daily Routine", which will be discussed in depth, later in this book. *Remember, all of the changes made followed a plea for help. Remember, my prayer was answered.*

And, with the answer, there was Hope!

A New Beginning

This new process, *(The Daily Routine),* began on July 15, 2005, when my new medication arrived. And so, it began.

One day there was a prayer, and the next day, there was a new direction.

There were two other very important things. Each day would preferably *start with prayer* and would *end with prayer.* This was not a direction that I could take alone. I needed, and still need, and will always need, *GOD's* help. That was, perhaps, the most important part of my daily routine.

For those people who are not comfortable with computers and charts, or statistical analysis, there is an easy way to accomplish many of the same things with manual graphs, which will be demonstrated later. The main idea is to get comfortable with looking at information in order to understand what is going on in your particular situation. The process of *writing down (logging) information* regarding an area of concern seems to be a true aid in *taking charge* of a medical challenge.

You Can Do This!

The Effect Of Advertising

As I searched for the root of my problems, other factors entered the picture. Not long ago, as I traveled highway 31 North, in North Central Indiana, I heard the radio. There were advertisements like, Big Mac is great, The Whopper is wonderful. KFC's chicken is Finger Lickin' Good, Long John Silver's Deep Fried fish is simply wonderful, and Hardee's Star Burger is out of this world. All of that wasn't on the radio, but part of it was. The rest were on bill board signs that I saw. And on and on it went! Whether I saw it on TV, or heard it on the radio, or saw it on a billboard along a highway, I was bombarded with advertisements suggesting that I needed to eat their wonderful products. Not only that, but, there were several restaurants close together, suggesting that any time I wanted to eat, they were there. After I arrived home, I heard & saw more of the same. I consciously turned the mental switch off, but, none the less, I heard, or saw, the ads. The next day, I was at a local grocery store, buying things that I simply had to have, when I saw Johnson's Bratwurst. Now I remember. The night before, I had seen it advertised on television. It was already in my hands and I remarked to my wife how effective their advertisement had been. She, of course, reminded me that she was not affected by advertisement. The truth is, we all are. We live in a visual society. The images we see make powerful imprints upon our minds. Most of the time, I was not even aware of _the powerful effect of advertising._ But, fighting this war forced me to take a look at a lot of things, and advertisement was one of those areas that I needed to address and do something about.

Part of the problem I faced is that the ads have changed from years ago. They are more effective. Just like the improvements in many industries, including the medical arena, there are major improvements in advertising.

Advertisements are shorter in duration, but that hamburger, or product, occupies the entire television screen, with the cheese melting off the side of the hamburger. Years ago, a man would be seen standing with the hamburger in his hand on a 30 inch tube TV. You would see the entire man, like Michael Jordan, holding his preferred hamburger. Not today! Now it's a 42" or bigger flat screen TV with much higher resolution. The hamburger or other product fills the entire screen! The imprint is made as soon as I look at it or hear it. Yes, I love hamburgers. I am an equal opportunity guy. I love them all! And, I love almost all kinds of food! Suddenly I was hungry, I begin to think about the next meal and that became or was my daily routine. Often, during the day, my thinking was "what will I eat next?" Day after day, week after week, and month after month it was "where will I eat next?" or "what will I eat?" Perhaps I should call "The Daily Routine", "The New Daily Routine". Let's not get carried away!

Does any of this sound familiar?

<u>Over-Eating</u>

Over the years, I had developed a love for food. By now, that's not news to you! The flavor was so appealing that I wanted the sensation to go on and on and on. So powerful was this feeling, that I would sometimes find myself looking over my shoulder at about ten in the evening, as I was making two bologna sandwiches or some other concoction. I should not have been putting that food into my stomach at that hour, or perhaps at any other hour. Now, a rational person should have known something was wrong. Yet, that urge to eat was more powerful than the thought "I should not be doing this!" None the less, I was drawn to eating to the degree that when I discovered that I was a person with diabetes, I decided to find my own way to beat the heat. The heat being the process of being a person with diabetes and yet still enjoying life. At that time, eating was a big part of enjoying life.

In 1998, life, to me, consisted of getting up early in the morning, slipping over to the local service station at 6:00 a.m., when they opened, just three blocks away, and picking up 3 wonderful, chocolate covered donuts, a large, steaming, black cup of coffee, and heading back to my home, where I ran a close tolerance machining business. I recently discovered that *this was news to my wife (the morning donuts and coffee)*. As the machining center would run, I would sit down, enjoy my coffee and donuts and plan the day ahead. I only weighed about 275 pounds on a 5' 11 ½ "frame. I had already lost almost 70 pounds, so what was the worry. Since I was not an active football player, something seemed wrong with those dimensions. I was fat, but, I was not going to say that. The truth is, *every day I was going to do something about my obesity*, but, for some reason, the day would pass, and *I would be faced with the same scenario the next day*. Have you ever had that feeling?

Deep down, I knew there was a problem. That's why I looked over my shoulder, when I made those sandwiches at 10:00 P.M. I did not want anyone to notice. That is why I was always going to do something about it, but there was always something else that interfered with addressing this problem.

Training & Observation

After I was told that I was a person with diabetes, and after taking training at a local hospital respective to nutrition and diabetes, I ran numerous checks on my system daily, and began to make some observations. I noticed that when my glucose was normal, the speed of blood entry into the test strip was faster. When it entered the strip slowly, I would usually have a high reading. That sent up a red flag. Suppose it had been high for a long time. If the blood entered more slowly, wouldn't that suggest that it was thicker? If it was thicker, wouldn't that imply that the heart had to work harder to do its job? If that was the case, no wonder persons with diabetes were more prone to have heart attacks, and strokes, and high blood pressure. *I also noticed that it was easier to get a blood droplet when my glucose readings were normal, than when they were abnormal.*

I have taken thousands of readings. *One of the most dominant observations was sample availability. As I mentioned above, using the standard stick method, when readings have been good, the sample has been easier to acquire. It seems that when the readings are normal to low normal, the sample simply is available.*
What that suggests to me again, is that my blood thickness is probably thinner, which might cause the blood to be closer to the surface of the skin which could make it easier to form a droplet to collect the test sample. Another explanation might be that being thinner, it could be easier to pass through a small hole in the skin. I have searched for clinical trials that would prove this hypothesis, but have found none. That does not mean that a trial has not been conducted. I am still searching other avenues. If a clinical trial has been conducted and it has proven that high glucose levels translate into thicker blood, then this could become a great training tool, because it would clarify why people who have diabetes are more prone to heart attacks and strokes.

When the readings are high, I have had to really work hard to get the blood droplet to come to the surface of the skin. *Sometimes, I have to adjust the lance to enter into the skin more deeply. That's when it gets a bit uncomfortable. More incentive to keep my glucose levels in check.*

Today, when I check my glucose, I rate the availability, the definition of the blood droplet, the glucose value and the speed of entry into the test strip. Of those (4) four variables, the most predictable is the availability, Yet speed was another indicator that was fairly predictable. Due to the fact that I take another medication which does affect blood thickness, I can no longer rely on speed as an indicator. I am looking for an organization that has already proven or disproved this hypothesis or an organization that will run a clinical trial in the interest of providing a great teaching tool for persons with diabetes, should it be proven that high glucose translates to thicker blood. It seems logical.

Building Resolve

As I began this new path, diet-exercise-and logging information, The Daily Routine emerged. It will be described in detail later. Nearly every facet of the process helped establish resolve. The most important element to build resolve was & is *prayer.* Prayer provides the foundation to stick with the plan. It takes a determined, planned effort, to overcome years of an established practice, during which the body is actively seeking certain sensations that simply make one feel good. Before this new path, eating for pleasure had been my goal. It was something I anticipated for a lengthy period of time. The more satisfaction I received from eating, frankly, the more I wanted. It felt good. It smelled good, and, it was good!

As I was feeling good, enjoying the wonderful aromas of great tasting food, I was expanding my horizons of weight and size, and creating a far more 'difficult-to-maintain' system.

I think the process of the *"Daily Routine"* has provided a balance of Physical Condition, Mental Awareness, Spiritual Strength and Perceived Well-Being. That has helped to build the resolve to *"Take a Stand"* and *"Stay The Course".*

Who is ultimately responsible for my health?

I am. Oh, the doctor can give me medicine, but what happens if all of my health cures rely solely on medicine, and not on my action or my behavior?

Every medicine I take has to be processed through the liver. Each one has negative side effects. The more medicine I take, the more chemicals that have to be screened. The less medicine I need to take, the better. Less medicine means less work on the system. Less work on the system means that I will reduce my chance of having problems simply by not introducing chemicals, which can have harmful side effects. The less medicine I need to take, the less cost for me and my country.

Who is ultimately responsible for my health? Me.

As I reviewed data over the first several months, there was less need for medicine. The evaluation of where my system is and where it goes as medicine is reduced is controlled by looking at information and making small adjustments and watching behavior without over reacting.

No change in medication should be made without the doctor's consult and consent.

I can have an idea, but the doctor is in charge and appreciates information supplied. It is the doctor that knows what I should take and how much. My information to the doctor truly helps the doctor help me. This has been proven over and over, as I have followed "The Daily Routine".

Who is ultimately responsible for my health? I am. What I see gives me Hope.

Make It Happen

As a manufacturing manager, in charge of a sizeable workforce, I posted a slogan in my office and on the manufacturing bulletin board. It was something that I started doing in the 80's, and I found that it reinforced the idea that if I wanted something to happen, (or had a goal), I had to do something. If I wanted a result, I had to provide a stimulus to achieve the result. It simply said, "<u>Make It Happen</u>"!

After I posted the message "<u>Make It Happen</u>", I called my staff into the office and explained what that really meant. It meant that we could not wish something and have it magically appear. It meant and means that we have to do something in order to achieve a desired result. Those people who ultimately got promoted were the ones who not only came to the office with complaints, but also came to the office with suggestions. Those suggestions involved doing something. Also, many times those shining stars did not agree with me. I appreciate thinkers, especially if they are the "<u>Make It Happen</u>" type.

If my staff wanted something to happen, then, they had to do something. Of course it had to be discussed, but the slogan "<u>Make It Happen</u>" became a popular mode of operation. Why? Because there was a lot of success. The people bought into it. So important was it that there were special awards to those who did something special. It might be safety, efficiency, or quality, but there was recognition attached to "<u>Making It Happen</u>". The recognition was a special company cap. Every time a new record was set, that person or crew received a gold star that was affixed to the hat. People tried to buy the hats and stars, but they had to be earned. When you looked across the floor, you could see a plant full of achievers.

This is another illustration, (even though it was my idea as a plant manager), of taking something from the industrial setting and applying it to my personal life.

In my case of fixing obesity, "<u>Making It Happen</u>" occurred as a result of answered prayer. That was the <u>first thing that I did</u>. <u>I prayed for an answer!</u>

First, on July 14th, 2005, the prayer was a stimulus. Then, the next day, July 15, 2005, the ideas emerged to provide a daily routine. I was not responsible for the ideas. They just seemed to be there. Then, there was a focus on <u>The Daily Routine</u>, and then there was achievement of the desired goal(s). *<u>Your focus and your goal are not always the same (to be explained later). Yet, there is a saying, "Your focus becomes your reality."</u>*

In order to "Make It Happen", something must be done. Seldom does a goal get reached by doing nothing!

"Make It Happen".

Cause & Effect

The cause is sometimes directly related to our focus and the goal is often related to the effect. For example, I want to lose weight. That is the desired effect. In order to achieve that effect, I may want to focus on something else that will help me achieve the goal. What has caused me to weigh too much? Many factors are present, but eating too much, eating the wrong things, eating at the wrong frequency and eating at the wrong times have all contributed to this problem of obesity. It took a while to come to that conclusion. My focus, then, turns to the cause. By that I mean I want to spend my energy on the things that created obesity. (What should I eat? How Much, How Often & When Should I eat?) This becomes my focus.

Here it is in a nutshell. The effect was obesity.

The cause was several factors:

Eating too much, skipping meals, not eating regularly, not eating at the right times, and eating the wrong things! What do you suppose happens when you eat two bologna sandwiches at 10:00 P.M.? Is that the right food? Is that the right time? Is that the right amount? Does that fall within the right frequency? If I am going to achieve my goal, which is to lose weight, until I reach my normal weight, I had better focus on what caused me to weigh too much in the first place-(the causes). In order to do that, I need to identify the cause(s). I think I just identified many of the causes.

Now we are getting down to the root cause(s).

In terms of getting a handle on this, I want to equate Cause to Focus and I want to equate Effect with Goal.

If my goal is to achieve a normal, healthy weight-the effect, then my focus will be on doing those things which will help me lose the excess weight (On the cause(s)). Enter "The Daily Routine".

It is truly simple:

Focus on The Cause = Reach the Goal Effectively.

In essence, I want to be aware of the effect or goal, but I want to spend my energy on the cause or focus. Therefore, if a discipline will bring my weight into a normal zone, I want to focus on that discipline. In this case, "The Daily Routine" gets my time!

The Daily Routine.

Early in the process, my daily routine was as follows:

Morning	Noon	Dinner	Night
1: Prayer			
Read			
Scale	Glucose	Glucose	Glucose
Glucose	Systolic	Medicine	Intake
Systolic	Diastolic	Intake Food	
Diastolic	Pulse		
Pulse	Intake-Food		
Medicine			

2: *Record* The Data
& Some Other Variables that were added later were;
Exercise
Sleep
Stress
Coffee Intake

Liquid Intake
Solid Intake

Charts	Charts	Charts	Charts

3: *Evaluate* the Record

<u>*Prayer*</u>

Note....... The log is filled out in the morning and items like food intake, liquids, and stress, are logged from the previous day's activities.

This is the process.

When I start my day, the first thing that should happen is to offer a special prayer of thanks. Thanks for being able to wake up. Thanks for being able to get up. Thanks for the day.

The next thing I do is head for the restroom. I then empty my bladder and/or colon. Just do what's natural and do not go to any extreme measures. The point being, I want to be as light as possible within reason.

The next thing I do is to find a solid flat place and locate my scales. Place the scale in the same flat location each day and then turn it on. I step on the scale and get a digital readout. I make a mental note of the weight. Later, that information is put into the computer. I can also write the info on a piece of paper, if a computer is not available. Next, I take my glucose reading. In the beginning, I took glucose readings several times a day and especially just before meals. A total of over 4000 glucose readings were taken over a four year period. (The number of glucose readings went down almost every year). (5) Five years later, once every few weeks was sufficient for glucose checks, or so I thought. Once in a while, I had a day where I took several readings. If everything looked good, then I resumed with the same frequency of once every few weeks. The readings were recorded, once again, on the computer. Finally, blood pressure readings were taken and the same process ensued. Since weight control was, and still is, my most challenging goal, I took readings in the morning, before eating, and, I still record that information. (Every Day)

Now that the information has been collected and recorded, I analyze the information and look for trends. Trend data is provided in the chart section of my spreadsheet. I have created a chart that reflects the recorded information. Then I have a computer generated trend line that allows me to confirm the over-all direction, so that I can see progress or trouble. Is my weight gradually moving upward, going downward, or staying the same? The identical process occurs with blood pressure readings. (I can also see the numbers moving up or down, but the trend line is a great tool to ensure accuracy).

Once all the information is recorded, I also record several other items such as, the amount of sleep I got the night before, and how much food I ate. There are other things that I consider important elements, which may affect glucose or weight readings, including stress, medication, coffee intake, etc., etc.,.

There are several ideas included in "*The Daily Routine.*". One (Impartiality) is that by charting and recording data, I can become somewhat detached from the process. It seems to be a little less personal and it seems to be easier to be objective.
Two (Awareness) is that I am putting information into my brain, which allows me to be aware of what is happening. It is just possible, that with this information, things may happen mentally that can actually help. Many functions take place, and I am probably unaware of many of those functions, most of the time. Three (Resolve) is that it is possible that this process has helped me build resolve, or determination, and it may have also helped with actual biological functions to aid in weight reduction, blood pressure management, stress, and glucose control. This is hypothetical, but the fact remains that my system currently needs less assistance. My brain is seeing more data and remarkable stability is being realized. In effect, I am doing my own advertisement (on myself), and, it seems to be working.

Impartiality

It is important that I *not be too concerned with measurements or readings at the time that I take the readings*. My focus has got to be on collecting reliable information. If I decide to fudge a number, because of a negative result, it defeats the entire purpose of collecting information. *Data has to be reliable*. There is always a certain amount of measurement error. If a person wants to truly improve a condition, then being honest and focusing on real data makes it much easier to evaluate the item of concern. This process may provide a better way to select accurate options. Case in point- I purchased a glucometer that had much less expensive strips. The end result, however, was that the data was not very credible, because there was too much variation in the readings. On the same sample, I might see as much as a 20 or 30 point difference. That was excessive. The end result was that I quit using the meter, because I could not rely on the results.

Here is what happens. If I monitor my glucose levels for 3 months or for 6 months, and I think they are in a really good position, and it turns out that my levels are much higher, I run an increased health risk and I have wasted my time reading, recording, and evaluating the information. The money spent on materials to take the readings has been wasted. On the other hand, realizing that data collected was not accurate, I quickly switched back to a more expensive, and reliable test meter and test strip. This provided good data, which was borne out by the A1C test. That test showed me at 5.6 on the scale, which is very good. There were no surprises. My health status was improved to the degree I expected and both the physician and I were confident that this would, and will, continue.

Therefore, be impartial when collecting information. Worry about the information only after it has been collected accurately, and only if there are disturbing readings or trends. Then do something to make a correction and stop worrying. *Make sure to keep your doctor up to speed with your information and seek his or her guidance as you establish control and capability.*

Be impartial.

To clarify, if I have an unusually high reading that is in the danger zone, which has been established by my doctor, I will make an immediate call to the doctor, if that is the arrangement with the doctor. That would take place if this reading were abnormally high or abnormally low, and in the danger zone. The other option might be to take a prearranged step, like a glucose tablet, if that was the recommended procedure.

I have to emphasize that worry is an enemy, but, knowing when to contact your physician is something that needs to be worked out with the doctor.

Be impartial, don't try to influence the readings, and DON'T WORRY! There is <u>HOPE</u>.

<u>Evaluate the Readings & The Meaning Of Variables</u>

Evaluate the readings, once the readings have been taken and recorded. This should be done on a daily basis for items where control is a problem. The frequency should be based upon the element in question. There are two types of variables. An <u>independent variable</u> is a thing that may affect a <u>dependent variable</u> or an item of concern.

An <u>Independent Variable</u> stands alone. It is not affected by other variables. Solid food intake, liquid intake, and exercise are examples of <u>independent variables</u>.

On the other hand, weight, glucose, or blood pressure, are <u>dependent variables</u>, and can be items of concern and can be affected by <u>independent variables</u>, such as food, liquid, and exercise. I refer to them as <u>dependent variables</u>, because their value can be affected by <u>independent variables</u>. <u>Dependent variables</u> may need to be controlled by controlling the <u>independent variables</u>, such as solid food intake, liquid intake, and exercise. These three variables have a direct effect upon weight, glucose, or blood pressure.

Think about these two types of variables for a few minutes.

By the way, it is not necessary to know the terminology of Independent Variables vs. Dependent variables to succeed with "<u>The Daily Routine</u>". This is simply a little more information that can be useful, but not necessary to know or totally understand.

Following up on variables, weight, for example, should be read and recorded once a day, if weight is a concern. It is not necessary to do this several times a day, but, if a person wants to do it several times a day, that is fine also. In some cases, I record weight at different times of day. Glucose, on the other hand, needs to be understood. In order to understand glucose levels, a person might learn about the Glucose cycle and understand whether the reading taken is at the bottom, top, or middle of a cycle. Glucose levels tend to move up and down during the day and night. The direction depends upon food intake, stress, exercise, etc. These things like food & liquid intake, stress, and sleep are a few of the variables that affect weight, blood pressure, and glucose readings. I recommend as many as 8 to 10 glucose readings in a 24 hour period at the beginning, in order to understand what is happening in the blood stream. Sometimes, that may not be possible to do. That can be reduced to once a day or even every other day or less, so long as one has established control and the reading is taken at a good, representative time of day. As a type 2 person with diabetes, I prefer to take a reading at THE ONE TIME OF DAY, when it will likely be at its highest-before-meal level (worst case scenario). I take my readings before eating, and generally find that early in the morning gives me the best idea of what the day will be like.

I have coined a term I call *Glucometric Directional Inertia.* What I mean by that is this; during the day, glucose will move up and down. It takes time to reach a peak, or a high level, and then start down. It takes time to reach the bottom level and then flatten out and then start moving up again. Somewhere between the high and low is an average for the day. When I take my readings, I can predict, based on thousands of readings, about when I will reach a low and about when I will reach a high.

I can predict that I will be around 90 at 8:00 A.M. and that my glucose will be slowly dropping. As soon as I eat, the glucose will begin to rise shortly after I have eaten my meal. At some point, later in the morning, it will reach a peak and then begin a downward movement again.

The direction of movement is what I call *glucometric directional inertia. (I doubt that the word "Glucometric" exists. It refers to glucose behavior) (Further research reveals that Glucometric is a valid word).* When a reading is taken, which direction is the glucose level moving? Is the glucose level going up, or down, or has it reached the top or bottom of the cycle?

Do you have to know that? No. It is simply a help toward understanding your system, but it is not absolutely necessary to know the direction. By knowing your system well enough to predict the movement, you may be able to avoid taking a glucose tablet or putting something in such as orange juice to bring your reading up. It is simply an added tool used to manage diabetes.

It had been six months and I had established glucose control, and anticipated losing another 10 to 15 pounds. As a result, I continued to take 4 glucose readings a day, until I reached a stable level of weight. Then I anticipated that my readings and medicine should be known factors. By then, I should have been able to get a good idea about my glucose levels with only one reading a day. It took a long time to get true control.

This has been an expensive process. The medicine, test strips, and meters all cost money. It could have been far more expensive, however, if I had continued to be overweight. My prayers were answered.

Respective to evaluating the readings, I look for averages, lows, highs, freaks, ranges, and standard deviations. The charts and printouts usually provide all of that information, so that I can evaluate the behavior of the variable and address areas of concern.

When I take readings over a period of time, I am looking at pre-meal (or before each meal) readings. I want to identify the highest reading and the lowest reading and the average reading. The range is the difference between the highest and lowest reading. It could be related to a day, week, month etc. The range is directly related to a term known as "Standard Deviation" or "Sigma". To be effective with this system, you don't really have to know the term "Sigma" or "Standard Deviation", but you do need to be aware of the highs, lows, averages, and range. That information can all be established in a manual chart; however, it is much easier to have a computerized spreadsheet so that the calculations can be done automatically.

Again, if you are not comfortable with spreadsheets and statistical information, you can simply record and run manual charts and you should get the same effect.

I want to spend a little time on evaluations to give additional insight. When I first look at a chart, especially a line chart, I want to be able to quickly see the safe zone or target area. Additionally, I want to be able to see the caution area and the danger area. In effect, I want to quickly see where the readings are over time. Again, I want to stress the importance of looking for trends. I am a person with type 2 diabetes. I purposely attempt to not influence or be influenced by any single reading. I do note the cause for disturbances (abnormal high or low readings, if I know the cause). Typically, for glucose, I look at 65 to 130 as being the target area. 55-65 is the low caution area. 131 to 180 is the high caution area and anything over 180 is serious and regarded as dangerous. Anything below 55 is also regarded as very serious or dangerous. These zones, normal, caution, and dangerous, must be set by your doctor with you.

In general, my problem, as a person with type 2 diabetes, has been readings that have been too high. These parameters are for me as prescribed by my physician. When I look at the chart, I expect to see normal variation. I want to insure that most or all of my readings are in the target area (65-130). I look for trends or patterns. What is happening with the average? Is it moving up, staying the same, or moving down? Do I see systematic variables where several readings fall conveniently at both sides of the nominal line, one reading on one side, the next on the other (which is not normal), or do I see random behavior? Do I see radical readings that are going past the control limits? For this application, control limits are the high and low number of each zone. The normal or safe zone, the caution zone, and the dangerous zone have been described. For the normal zone, the high number is 130, and the low number is 65, in my case. The same applies for the caution zone as set by your physician. The high number for me is 180 and the low number is 55. The danger control limit is anything above or below the high and low number of the caution zone.

True control limits are set based on readings that are taken, but for this application, we can use modified control limits which do not vary and which will give us what we need to move forward and to make sound decisions regarding where we stand with our glucose readings.

Do I see normal distribution or are the readings skewed? Assuming the vast majority or all of the readings are on target, if I see a decline in the average and if that average is crowding the bottom limit of the target area, I want to look at several factors with the emphasis on medication reduction. For example (It's March of 2007 as of the entry), 10 months into the study, this would be about May, 2006, after several reductions in medicine, using the above guidelines, the glucose charts showed a significant move toward the bottom of the target area. I studied this trend for several weeks. In consult with my doctor, one medication was eliminated entirely and within another week, 25% of my daily dose was eliminated in another medication. This was tremendous progress. Again, this was coordinated with my doctor. Based upon the analysis at that time, I expect to make further reductions, as my system becomes more efficient.

On June 26, 2006, a little longer than (11) eleven months into this process, all medication for diabetes was dropped, with the exception of Metformin. I had hoped that all the respective medicine would not be needed, but additional studies proved that I still needed one pill a day to maintain control.

Remember, I had been taking (5) five pills a day for diabetes in order to keep my glucose levels close to normal. That had begun on July 15th, 2005. The reduction in weight, as I changed several things regarding my eating habits really helped the over-all problem with diabetes, and what I anticipated actually came true. I had contacted the doctor at the beginning of "The Daily Routine", and told him that I expected to need less medicine, and that is exactly what happened.

Documenting readings and placing them into a graphic format allowed me to quickly see what had happened and what was happening at that time. The behavior of an uncontrolled system heading into a dangerous direction was reversed. Instead of taking more medicine to help my system, medication was being reduced and/or eliminated.

Remember, everything began with prayer on July 14th, 2005.

Through the use of information put into a graphic format, I have been able to see & understand my particular system and identify problems and correlate problems for cause.

With that information, new courses of action were taken. Best of all, the forecasts made in writing to my physician in July, 2005 began to become a reality almost immediately. <u>He was one happy doctor, & I was and am one happy patient.</u>

Anticipation

<u>Anticipation</u> has been a key factor. Again, this is hypothetical. In July, 2005, I *anticipated* changing my life style. I *anticipated* changing the food that I ate. I *anticipated* reducing my glucose reading variation. What that means is that the high and low readings would become closer together. I *anticipated* reducing my glucose average. I *anticipated* reducing my glucose reading standard deviation and I *anticipated* a reduction and a possible elimination all medicines.

In July, 2006, control of diabetes continued. Four pills a day were successfully eliminated, which was the total prescribed Daily dosage medication / Glipizide in Early July, 2005. I was, and still am, off that entire prescription, since May 12, 2006 and I ran an average of 93 for the two week period prior to July 11, 2006.
Additionally, for Metformin, a reduction of a whole pill a day to ¾ pill a day to 1/2 pill a day to ¼ pill a day became effective June 26, 2006.

I anticipated that by July 11, 2006, I would no longer require medicine to control my diabetes. After close evaluation over several months, I was very stable taking one Metformin pill a day for diabetes. Much better than 5 pills a day! It takes a while for the total effect of medicine doses to take effect. Metformin takes about 30 days.

Even though I anticipated the elimination of five pills for all medication for diabetes, four pills per day were successfully eliminated. I still require one pill per day as of June 6, 2010.

That was a major accomplishment for which I am ever so grateful.

Anticipation is supported with letters to my Doctor on July 25th, 2005, September 24, 2005, June 21st, 2006, and September 21, 2007. They are included in the section entitled "Keep The Doctor Informed". Each of those letters consults with the doctor regarding the process being used, i.e. "The Daily Routine". Those letters are loaded with anticipation with regard to medication reduction, weight reduction and improved glucose control. These letters also included stated goals and were supported with data and charts that were presented for his evaluation. There was an expectation of success toward a healthier, stronger me. Included in the letters was Hope.

Thanks to answered prayer on July 15th, 2005, desperation was replaced with positive Anticipation and Hope.

Prayer II

The danger of daily routines is that they can become just that. A daily routine can become a regular, frequent, activity with little originality. Prayer, on the other hand, should be done daily, but each prayer needs to be special. After all, we are talking to the power above and beyond the universe. GOD has already given me something very special. Now HE has added more. HE has given me a second chance at a full life.

Each prayer ought to include time for listening. Each prayer should be given the best time. It's important that each prayer is special.

Don't let prayer become simply a *go-through-the-motion* prayer. It needs to be one of meditation, sincerity and humbleness.

GOD is at work and HE deserves our best time and best thanks. The first fruits should belong to HIM.

"The Daily Routine" of prayer should not be a routine prayer. It needs to be original and sincere.

Prayers don't have to be audible, but they do need to be original.

Success

There is nothing like success-Success Breeds Success.
Now, let's go back in time.

Five Month Evaluation - December 12, 2005

On December 12, 2005, I visited my doctor for a <u>routine checkup</u>. That was <u>(5) five months after the new path began.</u> The doctor was absolutely upbeat as he reviewed the latest data - (Success). When he checked my weight, he noted an 18-pound loss from 229 lbs on September 26, 2005 to 211 lbs, on December 12, 2005, less than three full months since the September appointment-(Success). Things like cholesterol and glucose levels were absolutely great-(Success). Finally, after viewing the data for a few minutes, he looked me in the eye and said, "You deserve a Gold Medal for what you have done"-(Success). I thought, the real truth is, *GOD* deserves the medal. I am reaping benefits from answered prayer-(Success). There is no way that I could do this alone without either guidance or help, or both, from *The CREATOR*. I know that God sometimes uses people. I felt that this man and his staff had truly been doing *GOD's* work, when they repeatedly told me that I needed to lose weight in order to establish and maintain control over my diabetes and blood pressure problems.

The previous (5) five months (from December 2005 back to July) had been a new direction for me. Many first time elements were now in place. This was the first time I had eaten (3) three or (4) four healthy meals a day on a regular basis in decades (Success). It was the first time I had eaten small meals regularly-(Success). This was the first time I had eaten meals without bread or potatoes or meat-(Success). It was the first time I had a conscious, deliberate plan to take control of my life through better eating habits-(Success), and the first time I realized that I had lost a good portion of my life, before I made this change. I never realized that I had lost a lot of my life. For example, today, I can trot across the back yard carrying a 2 x 4 and never give it a second thought. At the age of 64, I felt much younger. I began to think about this, when I was on the roof of the storage building. I had designed and built it, and while I was on the roof of the building, installing the roof panels on my knees driving hold-down screws with an automatic cordless driver, I knew something wonderful was happening. There is no way that I could have managed that activity in July of 2005 weighing about 250 pounds. That is when I began to realize what had happened. Over many years in the past, before changing to the new path, I had gradually lost part of my life, and never even knew it. How could this be? The truth is, it happened so slowly, that I never realized the penalty I was paying for the enjoyment of eating wonderfully tasting food.

The fact is, now, part of my new life is simply avoiding great tasting food. The fact is, today, I still have a desire to eat too much, whenever I eat good tasting food. So, the question begs itself, why eat it?

It was nearly (6) six months, since the change(s) had been implemented. I still loved food, but I avoided eating bread, potatoes, bacon, sausage, and ham, though, occasionally, I did eat red meat. It was always lean. I may always have trouble with control, when eating delicious food, or, I may gradually establish control, where I will be able to eat in moderation. Eating in moderation is much less problematic, when I eat foods like spinach, lettuce, green beans, zucchini and/or tomatoes. These foods are nutritious and yet don't taste so great that I want to have more. Focusing consciously on eating small amounts (4) four times a day is much more easily achieved, when eating foods that are good for you, but not necessarily great tasting. This is a big part of the learning process that took place, during the first 5 and ½ months. Now, combining this realization with data input and analysis continues to reinforce the resolve to continue to live a healthy life.

How often have I had the thought, I will lose weight today, and I will not over eat today. Then I realize, at the end of the day, I failed miserably. Now, I can think about *Success!*

Success Breeds Success.

Success is a true motivator.

The Wind In My face

In 2006, at about 200 lbs, about 130 pounds lighter than I was in 1995, I stepped onto the basketball court, <u>alone</u>, and moved to the basket. It had been a long time, since I felt that much wind in my face from movement on a basketball court. The feeling was, and is, great. I was lighter than I had been in years, I felt no pain and experienced the joy of playing and shooting the ball. Even though I did not step into a one on one situation, I felt the need to play.

After 45 minutes, I stepped off the court, knowing something special had been given to me. I left the court, not because I was tired, but because of the concern for pushing the circulatory system too hard. It was, and still is, tempting to stay out and continue to move with intensity, but, that should wait for another day.

Feeling the wind in my face was, and is, a thrilling sensation, and one that I hope never to lose!

Feeling the wind in my face is a reward that provides incentive to continue "<u>The Daily Routine</u>".

I have, indeed, been given a second chance.

Colon Status

As I have mentioned early in this material, I am a Non-Professional respective to health and or diabetes expertise. I accumulated about 1600 glucose readings during the first year. I analyzed the behavior patterns and I had a hunch that keeping the colon in a state of minimal material or nearly empty, was a plus for glucose and weight readings. I have started recording the number of movements daily. This is simply a hypothesis. Usually, there was one bowel movement each day.

The fact is, as I lost weight, the periods where I lost it quickly were usually accompanied by increased bowel movements. I am fairly certain that the increased bowel movements are a normal activity that doesn't require any conscious effort on my part.

Occasionally, the expression, "Green Apple Quickies" fit. It seems to be part of times when I lost a lot of weight quickly. As the charts show, I tend to sit at a certain level for a while and then drop suddenly. It seems that the colon had a mind of its own and would actually go through a house cleaning mode, during times when I lost weight quickly. This is just a hypothesis projected by someone with no medical expertise.

The Anniversary(s)

The First Year
As of the date, July 15th, 2006, in contrast to 2005, I only needed a small amount of oral medication to control diabetes! That day marked the first year anniversary of a new direction in life. It marked the first year of making changes that actually restored or gave back a portion of my life that I never knew I had lost! I must thank my *CREATOR*. I firmly believe that my prayers were answered. I also believe that I could not accomplish this alone.

The test then was to see how well the system maintained itself. During the next few months, with minimal medical assistance (from a diabetes point of view), I held my own. I still took blood pressure medication, but it had been reduced by 50%. I anticipated that I may be able to eliminate this medication.

The Fifth Year
It is now April 27, 2010. In a few months, it will be 5 years since starting this new direction.
I am still reaping the benefits of following "*The Daily Routine*." Over time, other items have been added to the daily routine. Control is still maintained, and, my glucose requirements are still 1 pill per day. I have a new target of 185 lbs. I have hit 190.8 several months ago, but, currently, I am running 200 lbs and dropping. The winter months seem to add weight, primarily due to inactivity.
As you can tell, I have continued to follow "The Daily Routine". I have managed to keep medicine for diabetes the same as it was in 2006, which is amazing. I still only require one pill a day, and the dosage has stayed the same. Hope still remains a constant part of this process.

Charts

The chart-Morning Glucose from May 28, 2009 through October 11, 2009- is the information that led me to drop daily readings and go to a frequency of one reading every two weeks. Bear in mind that, initially, glucose readings ran from 2005 through 2009, and during that time, as things got better, the number of daily readings were gradually reduced. As I analyzed the chart below, it showed that all readings were at, or below, 100. This was an incredible result. This went on for almost (5) five months. Combining this information with the results of the A1C test, I felt confident that control could be maintained by taking a reading every few weeks and then running an audit on some random day. I would randomly select a day where several readings would be taken. That would be the audit day. The audit hopefully is confirmation that everything is running within the safe range. During the audit day, if problems occurred, I would go back to daily readings, until control or predictability reappeared. These results must be well within a safe range. At that point, I should be able to go back to once a week or twice a month sampling (glucose reading).

Make sure to read the entire story, because later it will be determined that a reading every few weeks is too risky.

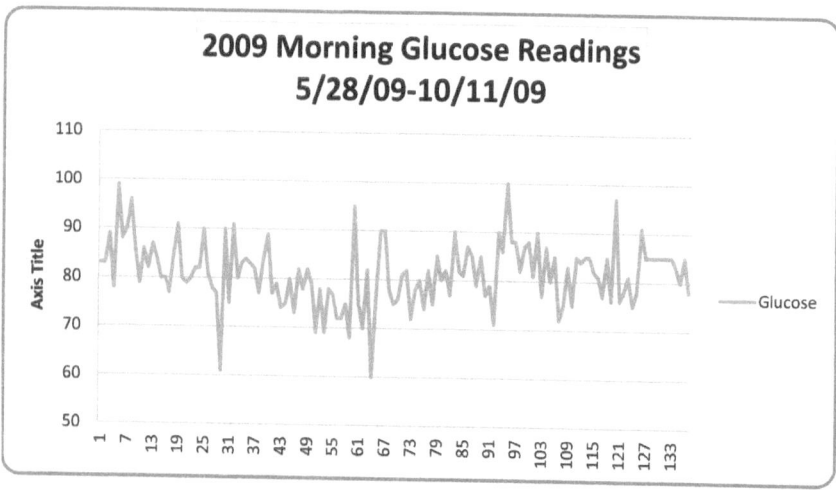

Great Readings

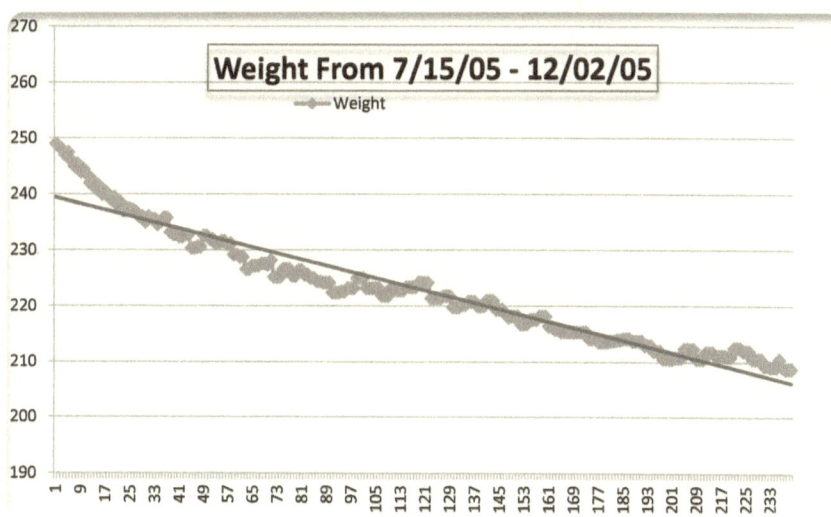

The chart above reflects the actual journey regarding weight loss, using "*The Daily Routine*" process. Weight loss charting actually began on August 22, 2005, a little over a month after I began charting my glucose levels. I backed up the data to the reference weight of 249.4 lbs, which was the weight on July 15th, 2005. Earlier in 2005, I was about 260 to 270 pounds.

Close study of this chart reveals that it was not a total downward record. There were several times when weight went the other way. In fact, more data, over the years, shows that it might go up for a few weeks and then suddenly drop. The main thing is to *STAY The Course*! Keep on keeping on. *Stay with* "*The Daily Routine*."

The glucose chart on the page below is an example of recording glucose information. It is a success story that began on July 15, 2005 and continues into the present time of 2010. The variation in 2010 has been reduced considerably.

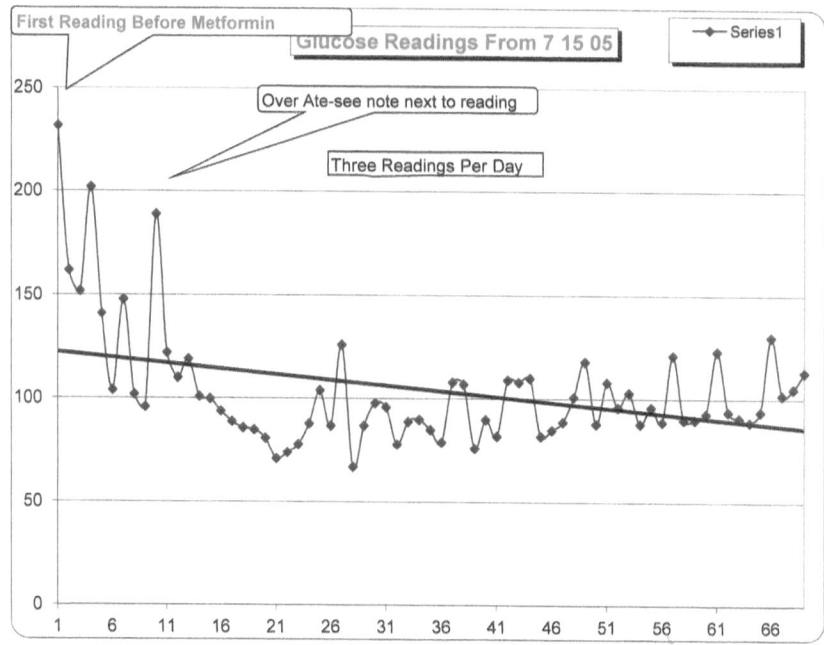

Glucose Readings From 7 15 05

First Reading Before Metformin

Over Ate-see note next to reading

Three Readings Per Day

Series1

For those who have type 2 diabetes, the foregoing information regarding mindset for recording information is vital. The chart has one long diagonal line that the computer generates. It is a trend line, and it is an important part of behavioral analysis. I am trying to keep the trend line in a direction which brings me into a normal glucose level, so the downward trend is important, until I reach the nominal 100 level. A new chart should be started as soon as normalcy is achieved. Your doctor can advise you on the range that he or she wants you to achieve. By recording the information and presenting it to the doctor, you can, in effect, help the doctor help you. The last part of this chart is approaching normalcy.

The thing to remember, when you look at this chart, is that it is an around-the-clock analysis. Some days, in the beginning, had as many as 11 readings, during the 24 hour period (that is in 2005). Today, in 2010, I may take a reading once in a two week period. The thing to remember is that the _A1C test really is the benchmark_ for glucose control. That test is performed, usually on a regular basis, and the frequency is generally established by your doctor. In my case, once every 6 months to once a year is adequate. The A1C level can change, and that is the reason I take periodic readings. Recently, I had a dental problem, and I saw a reading of 170. That was absolutely the highest reading I had seen for the year. It took 24 hours to find the cause, but as soon as the dental problem was corrected, the numbers dropped back to the seventies, eighties and nineties for the morning checks. Problem solved. I can now predict that the next A1C will have good results.

Today, in 2010, I can expect to see readings from 70 to 95 in the morning. In the beginning, morning was the worst time of day. Now, it is one of the best times of the day. What that means is this. If I want to really see how my day has been, I need to find the highest reading by time of day, before meals, and run my check at that time. If the highest reading generally is at 9:00 p.m., and I am ready to take one reading a day, then that reading should be taken at 9:00 p.m. If that reading is within the target area, then the entire day should have been a good day.

When looking at the chart, since I had been running too high for a long time, when I began to get back into a normal range of 70-120, I often felt light headed. That was especially true, if I hit numbers from 70's to the 80's. Even though those numbers are in the normal range, I felt terribly weak and wobbly. Sitting down was usually this first thing I did. That light headed feeling is a bad feeling and often, new persons with type 2 diabetes will nearly panic, and in many cases, the first corrective action is, "I need to eat something". Initially, that was me. Here I was battling obesity, and suddenly, "I needed to eat something"? I don't think so! That is a counterproductive response. So, what choice did I have? A friend led me to glucose tablets and as soon as I found out how effective these were to restore balance, I purchased a supply at a local pharmacy and found that I was able to get back on course without adding a lot of weight to my already heavy frame. I would simply take a glucose tablet and, in minutes, I felt good.

"Staying The Course" allowed me to get used to those numbers. While I was adjusting, any time I felt light headed, I would check my blood pressure and glucose level. If I was on the low side of normal for the glucose level and normal for blood pressure, I would then take a glucose tablet, which would quickly bring my glucose up, but still keep it in

the normal range. It took months of patience to get to the point where 70's and 80's felt normal. After several months, the lightheadedness disappeared. My guess is that when I got into the lower sector of normalcy, I was simply not used to that. I suspect that blood flow was better at the lower glucose levels and circulation was probably reaching areas more rapidly or more effectively, and I had to adjust to the change.

If you follow the chart closely, you will see that I noted the cause for abnormal readings. Usually it was food related or stress related. A few times, I simply could not find a reason, but over time, those instances of not knowing are really what caused the disturbance to become fewer and fewer.

Working with the doctor, there were medicine dosage reductions, which affected both glucose and blood pressure.

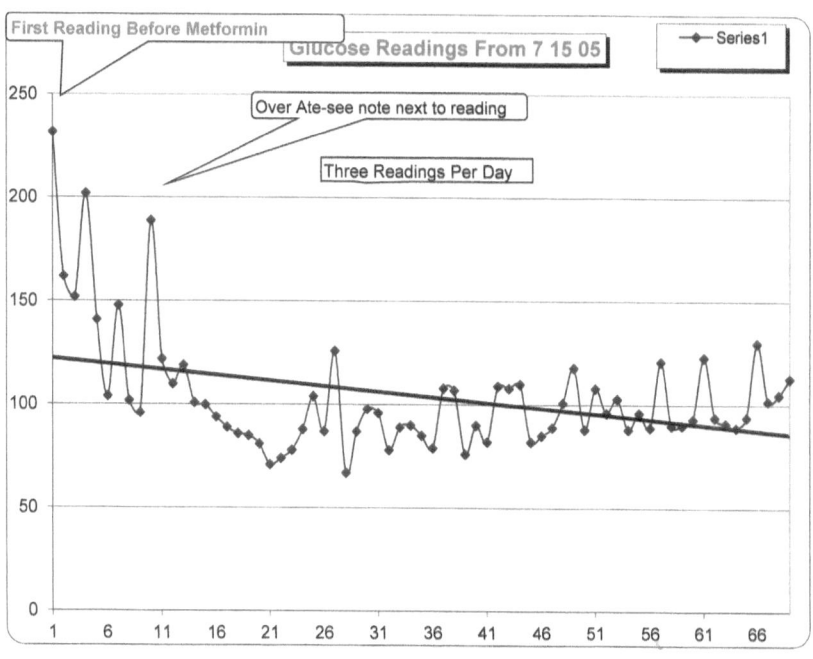

Glucose-Hypothetical-Manual

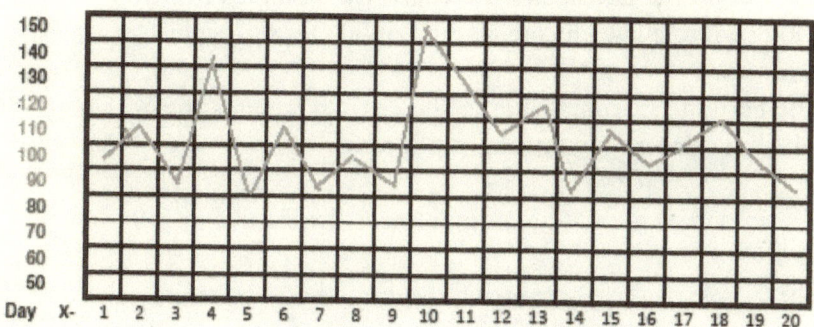

Glucose-Blank-Manual

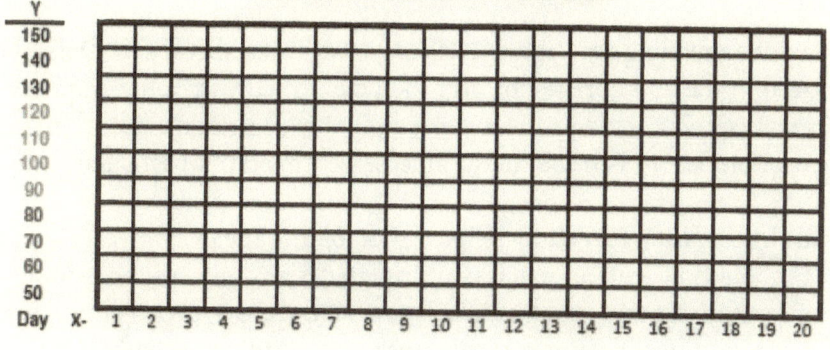

Glucose-Blank-Manual

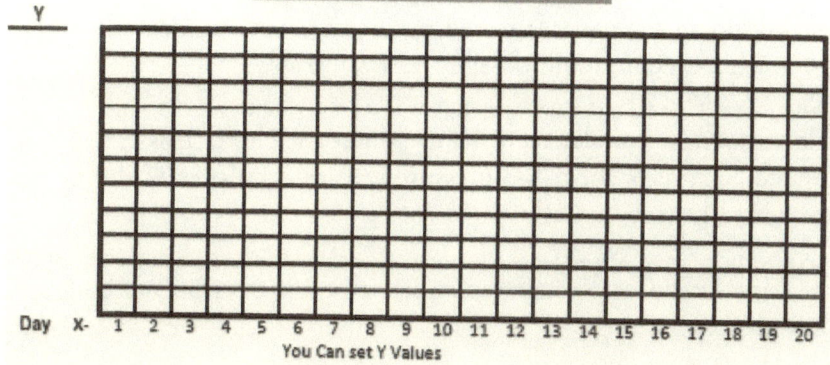

You Can set Y Values

Manual Charts

There are three manual charts on the previous page. The first chart is a sample Glucose chart, or hypothetical chart. In the <u>Y</u> axis, that is the column on the left side of the chart, the numbers run from a high of 150 down to a low glucose reading of 50. These are glucose values.

The bottom horizontal line of the chart represents the Y value of 50, which is dangerously low, in most arenas.

The second to highest horizontal line is the Y value of 150.

The X axis, at the bottom of the first chart, represents the day the reading was taken. In this case, we are looking at a (20) twenty day period.

Day one's reading was about 104. Day two's was about 117. Dots are placed in the appropriate box and then connected with a line segment. As you connect the dots, over time, a graphic illustration occurs and a person can see the behavior of the glucose system on this particular study.

This information can really help the doctor and it can give you a great idea about how your system is working. In cases where I see abnormally high readings, I will usually make a note on the chart, giving the reason for the reading, if I know what caused the reading to be high. This information really helps the doctor also. The same is true of low readings. Meal skipping can cause low readings, sometimes. Accidentally taking too much medicine could possibly be a cause also.

It is a good idea to take the time to fill out the chart. This can also be done for weight or for blood pressure readings. Pulse rates can be put on charts like this, as well.

The Middle chart is a chart with the same Y values but without any daily glucose readings.

The bottom chart is a chart that you could put the values into Y yourself.

If you are running 180 down to 120, for example, and you want to get your readings into a normal range, you might want to set your initial chart to read from 250 down to 50.

You can purchase graph paper at stores that have a stationary section, and then set the values according to your situation.

The main advantage that this provides is that it gives you a picture of how you are doing. By seeing this information, it can help you make decisions about things which you can do to help improve or influence the next reading.

There are some people who just don't like computers, or who have not had the opportunity to own or use a computer. Manual entries, just like the one illustrated, provides a good snap shot of behavior. That is what is important. The ability to see what has happened and being able to see what is happening can help you influence what will happen. It can also be an asset to you and your doctor.

This kind of information, computer generated or not, can really help your doctor help you, and, it can help you help yourself.

This mode of operation can provide a foundation for <u>Hope.</u>

<u>Staying The Course</u>

Finding motivation, focusing on achievements, praying, spending time collecting information, recording that information, and then reviewing achievements all contribute to "<u>Staying The Course</u>". Sounds like "<u>The Daily Routine</u>"! <u>Success</u> has been a great motivator! <u>Gratification</u> from buying new and smaller clothes has been another factor that encouraged me to "<u>Stay The Course.</u>" <u>Lower costs</u> for food have been another factor that has encouraged me to keep on "<u>Staying The Course.</u>" Feeling good has been another thing that has kept me on the path toward "<u>Staying The Course</u>"! People are one of the best tools for "<u>Staying The Course.</u>" Anytime a person has made a major change by weight reduction, after being obese for decades, other people notice. They can play a large role. As I began to lose weight, many people commented and encouraged me along the way. Some were people that I knew. Others were people I had met for the first time. Even some of them encouraged me to write a book. It was some of those people who encouraged me to write this book. Because of them, I was optimistic and my journey was made easier. Comments were made like, "You have just added 30 years to your life!" Or, "You look great!" "What are you doing?" "Wow, you should write a book!" I heard comments like this frequently.

(5) Five years have now passed. It is 2010. I thank *THE CREATOR* for placing people around me, who encouraged me along the way. Thanks to HIM, I have been able to "*Stay The Course*."

Their encouragement gave me <u>Hope</u>. <u>Hope</u> helped me to "<u>Stay The Course</u>."

You Get Out What You Put In.

This is a concept that goes back for decades of time. It goes back to my childhood, and had probably been around for years and years, before my childhood. Basically, we get out what we put into our minds. If we spend a great deal of our time preparing to eat for pleasure, and then eating for pleasure, <u>our focus will likely become our reality</u>.

In short, basically anything that we spend time thinking about has an impact on our behavior. If I spend time thinking about good tasting food, looking at commercials, listening to commercials, and seeing other forms of food advertisements, I am likely going to eat too much and eat the wrong things.

In my case, there is something about eating fried, good tasting food that really makes it difficult to eat a normal sized serving. I have a tendency to simply eat too much!

On the other hand, if I spend time looking at effects from eating the right food, the right quantity of food, and the right frequency (= number of times per day), then I will likely get out something good relating to weight management. The something good that I am talking about is the weight chart. If the chart shows that I have done well, I am more likely to keep doing well by doing the right things. Eating the right food will almost always happen and along with that will come eating the right quantities of food. If you look at the weight chart dated 4/29/14-9/29/14, you will see what I mean.

All along that particular period, I looked at the progress nearly every day. It is a remarkable chart, with remarkable results.

That is an example of the concept; "You Get Out What You Put In".

Choosing how we spend our time mentally as well as physically can have a major impact on what we do in life. Spending time on "The Daily Routine" has been a huge help to reverse years of obesity and high glucose levels, so putting in something good has yielded a great result.

The same goes for almost every endeavor.

Now, my main focus, when I purchase food, is to buy low fat, low starch, low carb, and low sugar products. I am heavy on fresh fruit and vegetables.
Some thinking discourages fruit, because it can tend to raise glucose levels. In my experience, even though that may happen, the levels drop quickly back into the safe zone. There are other benefits from eating fresh fruit that probably outweigh concerns for elevated glucose levels.

The results of this process have been great!

I get out what I put in, and sometimes more! In my case, Hope has been an almost constant companion.

Smiling & Laughter

Smiling & Laughter, in addition to prayer, simply put me at ease. My stress level is lower and therefore, I am helping to control my glucose level.

Here is a real life experience example:

For years, professionals have said that stress can be a real problem for glucose control. For a person with type 2 diabetes, that's me, stress can cause my glucose to elevate into unsafe areas. This is what happened.

As I was monitoring my glucose levels, I found that public appearances elevated my glucose reading. This happened almost 100% of the time. It did not seem to matter whether it was a speaking engagement, public meeting, or a music performance. If I was there, my glucose would rise.

Functioning in stressful situations involving public dissent or conflict always caused my glucose to rise, if I had any responsibility in the event. These disturbances were recorded over several months, and I became aware that smiling and laughing actually helped reduce tension, and or stress, and truly helped my glucose control. Telling an occasional joke helped ease tensions too.

So, if you are a person with type 2 diabetes, keeping things lighthearted is a good idea.

Smiling and laughter work for me!

Carrying the Load-Stress

On one occasion, I was concerned about a friend who was having serious problems. My concern grew to a near obsessive condition. I was eating the same basic foods, the same amounts, and at the same time of day. Suddenly my glucose level went from about 100 to 175. The next day it was about 180 and the 3rd day it was 185. _I became angry_, because all the control tools that I was using were not working. The anger did not help either. In fact, anger probably caused my glucose to rise even more. Finally, I identified the problem. _It was me._ I had been worried about something. This was something that I could not control. A light came on and I really began to realize the importance of stress and how it could affect glucose control.

The night the light came on was bible study night! I was on my way to bible study, when I thought I knew the cause of my high glucose readings. After bible study, I went into the sanctuary alone, and prayed. I stayed there for quite some time, and when I got ready to leave, I knew the burden I was carrying seemed to have left. I just knew that the problem had been resolved.

You know what it is like to worry about something. There is an uneasy feeling that you just carry around. Well, after spending time in the sanctuary, all alone in prayer, suddenly, that heavy feeling was gone. It was as if someone had taken a huge weight off me. Well, someone did!

That night, those things were put into the hands of "*THE LORD*" and the very next day, my readings fell into the normal range. It was not just close to normal, it was normal.

There are simply some things that we cannot fix or handle. I learned something very valuable that night, & smiling and laughter returned, and my prayer was answered.

What was also interesting about this is that about a year later, in front of our congregation, I related this story in general terms. I never told the specifics about who I was worried about or why. That was personal to the person having the challenge. I did not ask if it would be okay to talk about that. I just knew that this person really needed some help and I was powerless to make the fix. When I left the pulpit, my wife told me, when I sat down, that she wondered why I was gone so long that night. She had never said a word to me about that night. I am very predictable and have a habit of being on time for almost everything. That night was a different night. It was a good night. It was a night that allowed me to learn much more about stress and glucose control. It was tangible, and it was recorded. And, it reminded me of what I should do, when faced with a situation over which I had no control, and over which I was really concerned. Put it the hands of *GOD*. He handled it and rather quickly. Things were and are so much better now.

The bottom line-get rid of the stress! If you can handle it, handle it. If you can't, take it to the source! And, don't wait for three days to recognize which avenue to take!

The end result now is, I try to recognize those things that I can handle, and those that I cannot. That event was a great learning experience. And now, my load is lighter. I also have a much better understanding of stress and the effect stress has on my glucose system. It is no longer just a concept. It is a reality.

Stress affects glucose levels!

"Don't carry the load" needlessly!

Paradigm Shift

The first exposure to this term was in Manufacturing. It came from Statistical Process Control, and was referred to as a sudden, major change in process behavior.

Online supports this notion, in part. Per Wikipedia, "The term "paradigm shift" has found uses in other contexts, representing the notion of a major change in a certain thought-pattern — a radical change in personal beliefs, complex systems or organizations, replacing the former way of thinking or organizing with a radically different way of thinking or organizing." "Reference Wikipedia 2014".

The above definition comes from Wikipedia as one of the many definitions regarding the term "Paradigm Shift". In my story, this definition is absolutely true. This refers to a major change in my thinking and in my behavior.

It is 2010. This is a tough task. *It simply means making a major change or shift in behavior.* In my case, over eating, not managing my glucose levels, and not managing my blood pressure was a way of life. I enjoyed my life, but, I was not able to do the things that I can now enjoy. Making this change was difficult in the beginning. The first 30 days were the most challenging. As time went by, the challenge became easier and easier. Learning to say NO, to things that are pleasurable, was really hard. What gave me the best chance of success was prayer. Without prayer, I could not have accomplished this new path. It made the difference, and (5) five years, after walking this new path, I am still following "*The Daily Routine*", although the routine has been modified, as I have gained more control.

The truth is, I still run a chance of over eating. If I do not say no, mentally, to the volume of food available, I will likely eat too much. Many times, when we dine out, my wife and I are able to share a single meal instead of having two large meals.

Those who know me well can attest to this change. Refusing to eat certain foods or to eat at odd times is now a part of my daily activity, and it is predictable.

Without question, there is a major shift in behavior. It is a good shift! There is a "Paradigm Shift" from the days prior to July 15th, 2005.

Cost vs benefit

It is true that paying for thousands of glucose strips, over time, is costly. Over the 5 year period, I did buy several thousand strips. Today, I can almost go totally without any cost for strips. It took me a long time to understand my system. Someone else may not need to go to those extremes.
So, you could say that I spent several thousand dollars to get control of something that I never should have had to control, or over something for which I should not have lost control.

You would be right. Then, I look at potential costs for hospital stays, surgeries, and other potential medical problems. I could be talking even more thousands and thousands of dollars, not to mention the benefit of now having a fuller and more complete life.

The benefit exceeds the cost, without question. I have been blessed. And, with that I have Hope!

Taking A Stand

After years of failure, after being told that my physical situation was getting worse, that my pancreas had quit producing insulin, and after being close to the bottom, regarding my health status, taking a stand to do something was comparable to making a change, after someone put a gun to my head.

I simply got fed up (pun intended) with the status quo, and realized that what I had been doing for years, (Self Indulgence), was not only not working, but, could be causing things to get worse. That is when I put out the plea to GOD. It was July 14th, 2005. My stand started on July 15th, 2005 and continues to this day.

Sometimes, we have to reach a point of dire need, before we realize we need to take a stand. In my case, that was very true.

I took a stand, and am still standing, and it is great to not be in a state of despair.

And in place of despair, there is HOPE.

Motivation-The Importance Of Feedback

Motivation from feedback is a cornerstone of success. Feedback is information. This information is usually specific to some activity. In manufacturing, it is usually production efficiency expressed in percentages, or it can be safety or quality conformance. It can come from people, from reading data, from recording information, and from analyzing data. Motivation can come from people, attitudes, and focus. When I step on the scale, I will always round down the number, mentally. If I was 198.9 today and 199.2 yesterday, then yesterday I weighed 199 and today I am 198. This helps me continue to walk the talk or "Stay The Course." The Feedback motivates me!

People play a large role in feedback.

The recorded documentation can be used to help motivate me to continue on this journey toward self improvement. When I bowled, I watched the score and enjoyed striving to improve. There was honest feedback. There was always a target in front of me-the goal, and I was always able to see the results of my effort. Whether the results were good or bad, I still saw them.

(Feedback)

Now, suppose I went bowling, and every time I threw the ball toward the pins, at the last second, the pins would raise and then reset. I could not see the result from throwing the ball down the alley. After a while, I would simply lose interest in throwing the bowling ball.

Now, suppose that I threw that same ball down the same lane, and all the pins fell down each time I threw the ball. After a while, I would lose interest and not go bowling, because I could not see the true results of my efforts. I simply did not have good feedback.

Feedback is a big part of "*The Daily Routine*". It is a necessary component. It is important to get feedback, in order to know how you are doing, and, in order to fuel a desire for more improvement.

When I look at charts, usually line charts in my case, that is a very important form of feedback, and it usually happens every day. From the weight chart, for example, I can quickly see how I am doing. That feedback is a great motivator, which spurs me on to continue or change my activities in order to get the positive result I want.

Feedback is an absolutely essential part of motivation.

The Good-The Bad- & The Ugly

The good, the bad, and the ugly actually are three things (that I am guilty of) that relate to diabetes, obesity, and high blood pressure. *The good, the bad, and the ugly* are actions or results of actions that I took, after being told that I was a person with diabetes in 1998.

The Good 1998

Restricted Sugar-No food with more than 4 grams of sugar would be eaten.
Daily exercise became part of my regimen.
Cheese intake was reduced significantly.
I strictly observed medicine dosages.
I lost some weight.
I recorded glucose levels.

Took Nutrition Training
Received Diabetes Training
Established Short Term Glucose control
Analyzed Behavioral Charts
Research- I did a lot of research.

The Bad

I still ate some of the the wrong foods.
   Potatoes
   Carbonated Drinks
   Fatty Foods
   Bread
   Pancakes
   Red Fatty Meat
Large Meal Sizes
One Meal A Day
Skipped days per eating up to four days on one occasion
Plateau - weight loss. (Dropped to about 260-270 lbs and stayed there.)

Did not listen to the professionals
Quit Recording Data
Lost glucose control

The Ugly

Obesity continued.
The results became terrible.
Intermittent Glucose Control.
High Blood Pressure.
Horrendous Medical Costs.
   Supplies
   Medicine
   Doctor Visits
Limited Physical Capability.
The Loss of A high quality life without even realizing that I had a lower quality of life.

So much for the good, the bad, and the ugly!

Unfortunately, the Bad and the Ugly outweighed the Good and led me to 2005 where I reached a very low point in my life, medically speaking.

No News Is Good News

Hear No Evil, See No Evil, and Do No Evil. What this means is that if I don't hear about a medical problem, I don't see data like weight that is too high, and if I am not aware that I am doing something that is causing a problem, then, surely there is no problem. I truly did not want to see a problem. As long as the problem was not in front of me, surely there was no problem. In short, No News is Good news!

This was a big part of my daily life. There were huge problems looming, in more than one way. By ignoring information or not seeking information, I ended up with a potentially serious condition and remained obese for decades.

The fact is, as long as I didn't see information showing that I was in trouble, I did not have to face that fact. No news was good news!

The War

The name *"In The Trenches"* is a description of a series of battles that became a war. This was a personal war.

The war was a struggle. It was a struggle of gratification from eating food that brought pleasure versus eating food that was healthy. It was a war of gratification versus winning the war. *It was a war of gratification-Feeling Good versus Being Good.*

This enemy in this war was and is powerful. The desire to eat for pleasure is the enemy. It was so strong, that much of my life was spent in determining what good tasting food I would eat next.

The power of flavor was so strong that when I did eat, I always ate more than I needed, and, I always wanted more than I needed. I thought I ate what I needed, but, the need, at that time, was simply a need to experience the flavor that brought a feeling of joy. The key word(s) is, "Feelings Of Joy!" (not true joy).

Here is something to which you might relate. It isn't just solid food that I am talking about. Good tasting drinks like orange juice or other refreshments would have the same effect on me. Consider that a glass might be 12 ounces. If I drank two or three glasses, we are talking about one to two pounds in rough terms. Weight is weight. The body has to absorb it and shed it.

So this war that I talk about in the past tense is still something that I must consider to this day. Today, I am winning the war. I am running around 183.0 pounds as I make this entry on September 27th, 2014. This is definitely the best weight that I have reached since beginning this new path. I have to keep alert, in order to continue to win this ongoing war. I simply need to think about what I am doing, when it comes to eating food and drinking refreshments.

The good news is, since I have regained much of my life, and am now enjoying so many things, I don't have to think too often about what I am going to eat or drink, until meal time is here. I am not consumed by the powerful desire that I was prior to "The Daily Routine".

With that in mind, there is Hope. And for that, I am glad!

A Focus Away From Weight Management & Toward A New Discipline

Much of this is referred to in Cause and Effect, but it is really worth repeating, so here goes.

The goal was to lose weight and then maintain the weight loss. In order to achieve that goal, the focus went to "The Daily Routine", starting with prayer. The by-product of following "The Daily Routine" was weight loss and weight management.

The main thing on my mind was to follow the steps. Pray, empty the bladder and or colon, hit the scales, take the glucose reading, read the blood pressure information, and then, record the data. After that happened, I analyzed the information. That was my focus.

In the beginning it was glucose oriented. Then later, the process included weight, and finally, the process included blood pressure. The same spreadsheet later looked at other possible variables such as sleep, solid food intake, liquid intake, coffee, stress, body temperature, glucose sample speed, sample definition, exercise, medicine dosage, citrus intake, and other things, like bowel movement frequency. (_pretty radical_)

This process became a mechanical process from the standpoint of collecting information, recording information, and then analyzing that same information. The emphasis was to look at trends over a period of time, such as weeks and/or months. This really helped me to become objective.

This process was somewhat radical or novel, but, it also helped me shift my thinking from immediate readings to longer term trends. Those pieces of information helped direct my daily activities. For example, if I was low on exercise the previous day, I might spend more time exercising the next day. If glucose readings were off, after a while, I would automatically adjust my solid and liquid intake the same day and/or the next day. The process allowed me to be more objective, and, it gave me a chance to combat the high degree of food advertising that was all around me.

In essence, instead of focusing on weight management, I focused on the process called "The Daily Routine".

The information I collected, with the exception of sleep (I recorded hours of sleep), was based upon a 10 point scale with 10 being the highest and 0 being the lowest.

Food intake target was actually 5, so that I would not eat too much or too little.

Food was eaten 4 times a day, although in the beginning, it was 3 times a day.

The values recorded regarding the 10 point scale were estimates. We know when we have had a stressful day. The number for a stressful day will be higher than on a day when there is little stress. On a day where there is little stress, I would record the number (5) five. On days when there was great stress, I would record a higher number. There are some days that are almost stress free, and on those days, I would record lower numbers. The most important thing is to try to be consistent with the rating.

By looking at all of the information, this became exciting, because I could see what was happening, and, I could also influence the result by modifying the pertinent behavior. *This process helped me become detached or objective.*

Sometimes, increased prayer might be the cure.

Improved weight management simply became a byproduct of the <u>shift in focus away from weight management and toward a new discipline or process called "The Daily Routine"</u>.

The second paragraph talks about maintaining weight loss. It has been (9) nine years. I have not only maintained the initial weight loss but have actually hit a great weight level recently that is the lowest, since shifting my focus from weight management to "<u>The Daily Routine</u>." With the continuing success over the years, I have <u>Hope.</u>

Time Investment

This process requires time. Every day, especially in the beginning, I had to be willing to spend about an hour a day, going through the process. Before starting the process, it is important for the reader to review this entire book. The reason for that is this: *This process will not be acceptable to some people!* The process is really designed for the person who is fed up with fighting the war every day, and losing nearly every battle. I refer to that as being "*In The Trenches*!" Whether it is obesity, or glucose control, or blood pressure problems, to go to this extent to bring about a change or paradigm shift, one must be willing to invest time and resources, and be willing to make a change. Sometimes, we have to be in a state of desperation, before we are willing to try something new or do the right thing. In this case, we must be willing to invest time.

After being on this path for so long, I know that I cannot be successful, even today, unless I am willing to invest time. Now, (9) nine years later, I do not have to invest as much time, as I did in the beginning, but, I still have to spend time following the process.

Since my primary concern is weight management, I do not have to purchase anything additional in order to read, record, and analyze my weight. That is a big plus!

One must be willing to trust *GOD* and pray every day for resolve.

Why spend time after nine years? The fact is, I get reinforcement(s), even today, by spending time following the process. Perhaps the second most important time investment is reviewing my weight chart. The decisions that I make during the day are often the result of looking at where I have been, where I am, and where I want to go. I am reaching a point of wanting to maintain my current weight level. What I eat, how much, and when I eat are still influenced by what I see regarding my current and past weight status.
By reviewing my chart for the last 5 months, that information remains fresh and it helps me to sustain the wonderful progress that I have made.

"The Daily Routine" has given me Hope! Now, if I start to head in the wrong direction, I know that I can have great results. I do not take the credit for this. I have been blessed!

I have Hope!

What Kind Of Price Tag Do You Put On Your Health?

There are, unfortunately, many people who pay thousands and thousands of dollars to correct or relieve a medical problem. A person failed to eat the right things. This person had type 2 diabetes. Ultimately, this person suffered an amputation. The procedure, the stay in the hospital, and subsequent therapy, cost thousands of dollars.

Another person suffered blindness, as a result of uncontrolled diabetes. There are many stories like these. Many of those same people, if they had a chance to do it over again, would take steps to prevent the loss, if it was preventable.

There used to be an advertisement regarding automobile maintenance. It went like this: "Pay me now, or pay me later." This referred to performing preventive maintenance by changing oil regularly to prevent early engine failure. The cost of prevention was much less than the cost of correction, or repair. For a few dollars, a person could have the car lubed and get an oil change and a new oil filter. That insured longer engine life. Failure to perform preventive maintenance almost always ended in major repair costs like engine rebuilds with new rings and valves, etc., etc., or even a new motor.

In people, add to that, the loss of the quality of life, and prevention wins, hands down.

Many people simply don't anticipate the agony of defeat. Now, I would much rather pay money up front to get control of a medical problem, rather than ignore the problem, and then suffer a huge medical cost, that could have been prevented. I speak with great authority on this subject!

In my case, hundreds and probably thousands of dollars were spent, after losing control. Again, that cost of regaining control, very likely, could have been prevented, if I had only followed the advice of the professionals.
However, in my case, it was, and is, *"Better Late Than never!"*

"The Daily Routine" is designed to identify and attack the root cause of many health control issues. It promotes a process, rather than a specific diet, or a specific medical procedure, or a specific exercise system. It promotes resolve, which has been previously addressed under the heading "Building Resolve".

So, what kind of price tag am I willing to pay for my health? I would rather pay an amount that protects and maintains my health rather than to pay the outrageous costs to repair a failed system. I would rather protect a good system or reacquire good health, rather than wait and then lose a quality of life, which might never, be regained.

In my case, I was given a second chance. Not everyone is so lucky. Not everyone is lucky enough to be able to make the choice to regain their health.

Building Resolve supports the idea of controlling costs by paying preventive maintenance costs, rather than not taking proactive measures and then having a major cost due to a probable, preventable health problem.

Putting money aside, the physical and mental experience of having a medical problem can be horrible. When you consider losing limbs, having heart attacks or strokes, becoming blind, which can all be related to diabetes, there can be tremendous suffering that might have been prevented.

Prevention is a far better option than repair.

So, what kind of price tag am I willing to pay for my health? The amount necessary to prevent a preventable condition, and then some.

"What Do you Or I Have To Lose?"

This question is really addressing the question of, "Do I want to choose "The Daily Routine?"

If we add the plusses and subtract the minuses, we not only have nothing to lose, but everything to gain. When I look at preventive measure costs as compared to costs for a stroke, a heart attack, surgeries, hospitals, doctors, nurses, therapies, and, when I look at the loss of the quality-of-life, due to not taking preventive measures, I am far better off to follow "*The Daily Routine.*"

In spite of costs to monitor, learn about and understand my system, I have had to be willing to <u>invest time</u>. And who knows? I may have actually <u>gained time</u>, as one of my friends said.

Knowing what I know now, I would do it again, (follow "<u>The Daily Routine</u>"), only sooner.

What Do I have to lose? Nothing-but weight, if I am over weight!

Is this a guarantee that "<u>The Daily Routine</u>" will work for you? No, it is not.

It is a fact that it has worked for me.

I now have <u>Hope</u>. That is a Blessing. I <u>Hope</u> you, too, are in a position to be able to make a choice! <u>Hope</u> is a powerful ally. I have <u>Hope</u>!

<u>The Labor Of Excessive Digestion</u>

Although *<u>I am not a medical professional in any sense</u>*, I believe that digestion, from eating large meals, puts a strain on the human body. By now, you realize that I make a lot of observations. Most of these are based upon statistical data that I have collected, recorded, and analyzed. Fatigue is not a variable that I have analyzed, though it could have been or still could be added to the list. There is no meter for fatigue, so it would be somewhat subjective, yet, like stress, I could apply a theoretical number, because there are some days that I know I have more strength, than others. This is a fact, because during part of my life when I lifted weights, there were days that I could lift more weight than on others. I am not the only person who has experienced that. My guess is that you have the same experiences of stronger and weaker days.

Getting back to the labor of excessive digestion and the fact that I think it puts a strain on our bodies, I also think that the bigger the body, the greater the strain on the heart. Consider the idea that a larger body has to be supplied with more blood. Regardless of size, the more a person eats, the more processing that takes place. Very likely, more insulin has to be produced as well as other things that pertain to digestion and system balance. *The end result is that digestion does require energy*. I think the more digestion that takes place, the bigger the strain on the vascular system. Glucose is produced, when a person eats. I think that during the production of glucose, the blood gets thicker. If that is true, then the heart has to work harder to pump the thicker blood through the body.

Therefore, it makes sense to eat small meals. Keep the system working efficiently with minimum energy to process food. This is what the professionals say, "eat small meals" and it makes sense!

The labor of excessive digestion-due to eating oversized meals is a hypothesis that is likely true. According to some sources, under certain conditions usually related to a disorder, digestion may cause fatigue. I think in cases where over eating is involved, it absolutely will cause fatigue.

Avoid Eating Great Tasting Food

To succeed in keeping intake at a minimum, as stated earlier, I avoid great tasting food. This (great tasting food) should be eaten sparingly. The problem with great tasting food is that I want more. So long as I eat food that tastes good, but not great, I have the upper hand with regard to the volume of food that I eat.

By selecting food such as fresh fruit, or fresh vegetables, I find foods that taste good, but they don't give me the powerful urge to over eat. If fresh food is not available, then packaged or canned food is my next alternative.

On the other hand, if I start the day with toast and butter, or any food that has a lot of fat in it, the flavor is great, and, I want more. Not only do I want more at the time that I eat it, but, I start looking for more of that great flavor, and start to think about the next meal.

Part of building resolve is centered around avoiding those foods, which are great tasting, or the foods that have high quantities of fat in them. There is a direct link to glucose control problems and fatty foods. For me, there is a problem with appetite and great tasting foods. I want more, when I eat them. Stay away from them! The trouble lies with wanting to find great tasting foods that are good for you. Well, when I do that, I want more. Eating more, even if the food is good for me, means that I have to process more food and this is a problem for me. I must simply avoid eating too much. My best situation is to look for those foods that are good for me, but, not great tasting. Foods that are laced with excellent sauces and spices are the ones that cause me the most trouble.

Fried foods, which are definitely bad for me, have a tendency to be over eaten. I will want either a large serving or another serving, because they taste so good. I, as a person with diabetes, am not supposed to eat fried food. The best thing for me to do is to refuse to eat fried food. And, most of the time, that is just what I do.

An example of a food that tastes good, but, I do not eat too much at a sitting is fresh squash, like butternut squash. It tastes good, but, for me, I seem to get satisfied quickly and I do not have the feeling that I want to eat more. It's just the opposite.

We are all different, so perhaps this may or may not work for you. The thing is, when you find a healthy food that is satisfying and helps with appetite control, be sure to make a note of that.

For appetite control, I just have to avoid great tasting food.

Allowing the Body to Seek It's Own Weight

This may seem like a strange idea. What I really mean is that if I follow "The Daily Routine", I will pray, empty the bladder, step on the scales, and Read, Record, and Analyze. I will eat at the same time of day every day, I will eat high quality food, and I will eat small quantities. I will eat 4 times a day &, I will control my diabetes and blood pressure. Be mindful that the last meal is usually the smallest also. The bottom line is that I will be providing the platform for the body to seek its own natural weight, instead of continuing to weigh far too much. I need to give my body a chance to reach the optimum size and/or weight. Using this philosophy, I don't get too concerned about momentary elevations in weight. What I really want to see is a trend that shows that my weight is being reduced over time or that it has leveled off into a safe area. There are times when the weight does go in the wrong direction, over time. That almost always occurs, when I get lax about following the process. When that happens, *I step up my focus on "The Daily Routine". (See Pg 43 and review the weight chart again.)*

On Sept 24, 2005, I wrote a letter to my doctor and made an observation, in the third paragraph. At that time, I had only been on "The Daily Routine" for a little more than two months. This was my second letter. The observation was,"The body seems to seek its normal weight". At that time, weight loss was significant, and I did not see the noteworthy taper in weight loss that I had expected, during the first two month period. This was a powerful observation and very surprising! As I have followed "The Daily Routine", taper did occur, but, it was only when I got close to my normal weight level that I saw this happen.

Looking at the weight chart dated April 29, 2014 through Sept 29, 2014, in the section entitled "Losing Weight", I see a great example in weight loss that has finally put me on target with my normal weight. That example also illustrates a wonderful, controlled weight drop that resulted in about 22 pounds over a 5 month period.

It also supports the notion that the body will seek its own weight, if I do the right things.

On the journey, reflected in the chart, there has been a substantial presence of HOPE!

Doubt

This is the opposite of positive anticipation. <u>Doubt is not permitted</u>! Part of the reason, for going through this process of "<u>The Daily Routine</u>", is to provide motivation, every time a small step forward is taken.

Success breeds success. Success breeds confidence. With confidence comes positive anticipation. <u>Doubt</u> is simply discouraging. <u>Doubt</u> affects our will to succeed, persevere, and "<u>Make It Happen</u>". <u>Doubt</u> provides a distraction and requires energy. I must keep my batteries as high as possible in order to succeed. <u>Doubt</u> requires energy and saps energy. I cannot afford to waste energy on non-productive endeavors! In short, I cannot promote failure.
Do Not <u>DOUBT</u>!

<u>With doubt, it is easy to predict correctly</u>. If I mentally think, "I don't believe I can do something" (that's <u>doubt</u>), and then not do it, it is much more probable that I will be right and not achieve what I started out to accomplish. I will have just promoted failure. Saying "I can do this and "<u>Make It Happen</u>" is more challenging. Without <u>doubt</u>, I have a much better chance of success!

If I want to be successful, <u>doubt</u> is prohibited!

Do not <u>doubt</u>! Instead, have <u>Hope</u>!

Medication

All <u>medication</u> must be strictly supervised by the doctor. Any changes in <u>medication</u> should be approved by the doctor *<u>prior to the change</u>*. Following the process led to <u>medication</u> reduction. By keeping the doctor informed and setting goals, <u>medication</u> was reduced, as I reduced my weight.

The <u>less medication</u> that <u>I need to take, the better</u>. There are fewer side effects. Side effects are almost always bad. Side Effects like nausea, headaches, etc., can be avoided by simply not having to take medication.

Keep the Doctor Informed-Letters to My Doctor

There are (4) Four letters to my doctor enclosed that embrace and reinforce many of the fundaments described in our introduction. We have included them, because they are documents which track a very important time, which is the inauguration of "The Daily Routine". That is to say that within (10) ten days, after verbal communication with my doctor, there was written documention provided which supported the verbal communication and updated the doctor so that he could help me on my journey along the new process we call "The Daily Routine".

These letters are presented with the exception of certain personal information. They include Hope, anticipation, goal setting, goal achievement, Humbleness, Time Investment, Awareness, Exercise, Feedback, Results, Motivation, Success, Staying The Course, Paradigm Shift, and Prayer. The main thing they illustrate is the need to communicate, consult, seek and follow the advice and directions given by the doctor.

They cover a time frame of the first (26) twenty six months.

The other thing that has been stressed is that this process is not a specific diet, nor does it promote any diet. So references to what I ate or did not eat are specific to me only. If you decide to follow "The Daily Routine", your food should be chosen by you and/or your Nutritional/Diabetes specialist or your doctor. As a person with diabetes, I must eat foods that are hi protein, low in sugar, low starch, low carbs, low fat, and unfried. Diabetes specialists and nutruitionists are good sources for consulting regarding food that is good for people with diabetes.

The main focus here is on the process.

Letter #1 (HOPE)

7/25/05 (Letter & Charts delivered to DR X)
To: Dr. X

Dear Dr. X

Thank you for Metformin. It has acted quickly and effectively. During the first (5) Five days, my glucose readings have moved from seriously out-of- control to in-control.

Here's the data. I am presenting (5) charts along with the individual readings. For the first (7) seven days, (3) three readings were recorded each day. Now, I am recording (4) four readings per day. My first reading was at 11:30 AM followed by a reading at 4:00 PM then again at 6:00 PM. Since I took my first Metformin Friday 7 15 05 at 11:30 AM, I kept the readings in the same order. Now I am taking readings at 7:00 AM, then 11:30 Am, and again at 6:00 PM and finally the last reading is at 10:00 PM.

I have changed my diet to be high in fresh vegetables, with a rule and no eating of any kind after 7:00 PM. It includes lots of fluids-mostly water, no bread or potatoes and very little meat. Fish and poultry are ok. I have had to eat twice at about 10:00 PM, because I was concerned that I might go too low. My results have been very good using this plan.

The end result is that the weight is falling off at an unexpected level. As you previously said, the weight loss will really help my glucose readings and other concerns such as Blood Pressure.

The info enclosed is looking at weight, sleep, food intake, stress, coffee, and exercise as variables that may contribute to glucose levels.

Within another week, I will monitor blood pressure and record it as well.

A good portion of my career has involved statistical analysis. I am using that background to analyze my own situation. At one point, for at least a month in 2002, my average glucose readings were 88 with a high of 105 and a low of 65. I am not certain where this process will take us now, but I think a spread of 65 to 105 would be a good goal.

In the meantime, until my weight stabilizes, I will likely need to take four readings a day, to insure that I keep my glucose readings in control.

Metformin is an excellent medication. I am certain that the baseline blood tests taken today will support this information.

I realize that I have been my own worst enemy, because I allowed my weight to reach a high of well over 300 pounds several years ago. I am confident that I will be able to reach 205 lbs in a short time. I did become a little concerned, because I actually lost nearly (3) pounds in one day, as the chart will reveal. Most of that loss was water. I also need to know if you want me to take any type of potassium supplement, while I am losing weight.

With regard to the data and charts, I am monitoring the average, the highs and lows, the range, and the ever important standard deviation(sigma) and correlating that data to Sleep, Intake, Stress, Coffee, and Exercise.

Your advice is being heeded.

You should be aware that your nurse, I think it was Nurse 1, and also Nurse 2, stressed losing weight. Both of those people are good communicators and, in my opinion, are doing an excellent job. I appreciate their genuine candor and forth-rightfulness. Please pass along my thanks!

Your help is truly appreciated.

Best Regards,

Richard Phillips

PS

I did injure my left heel again- just after seeing you the last time. This was caused by carrying an instrument while I was walking on a very steep slope. It is better, but it is very sensitive. I also have a swelling below the left shoulder that has been there for a few years. My previous doctor did not think that this was a serious problem, but, if you were unaware of this, I wanted to mention it.

Over all, I feel good, but am very aware that the new medication is driving my glucose where it needs to be. Any time I get into the low 80's, I feel uncomfortable. I believe that I simply need to get used to being in that area and hope that this will be the case.

Letter #2 HOPE
9/24/05

To: Dr

Dear Dr

This is a follow-up to the letter of July 25, 2005. I have just completed a two month controlled study of a new discipline, which is centered around a term I call, *"Eating For Effect"*. *This is a planned "Paradigm Shift"*. During this period, I have gradually lost 24 pounds. This process, "Eating For Effect", will continue, very likely, indefinitely. Some modifications will be made, after my weight has normalized. The following are key points;

> Cumulative Weight Loss History

> Systolic & Diastolic Chart History

> Blood Pressure & Pulse History

> Systolic & Weight Data History

These Four charts show a computer generated trend line, which reflects a gradual reduction in systolic and diastolic and weight trends, while showing a slight increase in pulse over the study period.

All of these trends appear favorable

Page three shows Average, High, Low and Sigma.

My concerns are as follows;

I predict a future loss of about 20 to 30 pounds, before normalizing my weight. Surprisingly, the weight loss has continued to be about 2.5 pounds per week. Although I expected a rapid reduction followed by a significant taper in weight loss, that did not happen. The body seems to seek it's normal weight.

As a result, I expect to achieve my initial goal of 205 pounds during the next three months. I also think that I will actually drop another ten pounds, before this process really levels off.

Here are other significant factors;

Intake	No Bread, potatoes, soft drinks (carbonated), red meat, or fatty foods.
Hi Intake /	Fresh Vegetables-Some Fruit Also Usually have Micro Eggs

Moderate Intake (Roasted Chicken- Baked Fish)

Frequency	Intake is Four Times A day (Includes a snack at around 8:00 PM)
Intake Size	small!
Glucose Reading Frequency	7 Times/ Day

Daily Routine (Preferred)

Morning	Noon	Dinner	Evening
Prayer	Glucose	Glucose	Glucose
Scales	Enter Data	Medicine	Blood Pressure
Blood Pressure	Intake Intake	Enter Data	Enter Data
Glucose			*Prayer*
Medicine			
Intake			
Enter Data			
Evaluate Charts			

With a continued reduction in weight, I need a plan of action respective to medication. I am confident that further reductions in medication will be necessary. _I need to know which medication(s) I should reduce as levels drop too low or what options you would suggest._

Regarding Blood pressure, I also need your recommendations.

With respect to medicine dosage options, these concerns are all good problems to have.

Both my wife & I have purchased bicycles, which will become a larger part of our daily exercise as weather permits. I have joined the local YMCA, which is being used during inclement weather.

We have made serious changes in our lives, and I think these will be permanent changes in thinking and behavior.

Perhaps the second most important change has been the investment of time to evaluate.

Richard Phillips
PS

Additional Charts and data will be enclosed showing the last two weeks, the last month and the entire study period per glucose readings. The next blood test will reveal dramatic improvement in glucose control. Three months of improvement will be complete on October 20, 2005.

Two meters have been used with the majority of data per the Bayer Glucometer Elite.

Your help along with Nurse 1's & Nurse 2's is sincerely appreciated.

Letter #3 HOPE
6/21/06

To:Dr

Dear Dr

This is a follow-up to the letters of July 25, 2005 & September 24, 2005. I have just completed an (11) eleven month controlled study of a new discipline, which is centered around a term I call, *"Eating For Effect"*. This is a planned "Paradigm Shift". During this period, I have gradually lost 50 pounds. The process, "Eating For Effect", will continue, very likely, indefinitely. My weight is nearly normalized. My initial target was 205 lbs. That has been achieved and I am currently running around 203 lbs. My low has been 199.2 lbs on three occasions. My new weight goal is 195 lbs.

To assist, during the past week, I have reduced my morning intake by 25% and the fourth meal intake by 25%. The loss of 2 lbs has been realized during the past week. In effect, I am eating just below maintenance levels and believe the new target will be realized within the next three months.

The same daily routing has been executed during the past (11) eleven months. It is outlined later in this letter as well as previous letters.

Although I am not certain, I think the A1C results should be better than my last visit. There is one item of concern. We took a trip to

California prior to the last blood test. With the time difference, I had trouble maintaining good glucose levels as the charts will reveal. Four factors, time differential-stress-lack of exercise-and food, contributed to the poor results. This lasted for one week. We were back home by 1:00 AM the same day of the test. As you can see, the glucose behavior normalized immediately.

Although this is speculation, I sense that eating provides a trigger for the generation of insulin and other polypeptide hormones. In essence, the system appears to be re-programming itself.

Data For Your Review,
     Medical Dosage history
     Glucose History
     Blood Pressure & Pulse History
     Weight Data History

All of these trends appear favorable

My concerns are as follows;

Here are other significant factors;

Intake	No Bread, potatoes, soft drinks (carbonated), or fatty foods.
	Hi Intake / Fresh Vegetables-Some Fruit Also Usually have Micro Eggs
	Moderate Intake (Roasted Chicken- Baked Fish)
	Nuts, Berries & Diet Ice cream nearly every day.
Frequency	Intake is Four Times A day (Includes a snack at around 8:00 PM)

Intake Size   small!

Glucose Reading Frequency   4 Times/ Day

Daily Routine (Preferred)

Morning	Noon	Dinner	Evening
Prayer	Glucose	Glucose	Glucose
Scale	Enter Data	Medicine	Blood Pressure
Blood Pressure	Intake Intake	Enter Data	
Glucose		Enter Data	*Prayer*
Medicine			
Intake			
Enter Data			
Evaluate Charts			

My Wife & I have made serious changes in our lives, and I think these will be permanent changes in thinking and behavior.

Perhaps the second most important change has been the investment of time to evaluate.

_____

Richard Phillips
PS

Two meters have been used with the majority of data per the Bayer Glucometer Elite.

Your help along with Nurse 1 & Nurse 2 is sincerely appreciated.

Letter #4 HOPE
9/21/07

To:Dr

Dear Dr

This is a follow-up to the letters of June 21, 2006, July 25, 2005 & September 24, 2005. I have just completed a (26) twenty six month controlled study of a new discipline, which is centered around a term I call, *"Eating For Effect"*. This is a planned "Paradigm Shift". During this period, I have gradually lost about 60 pounds. The process, "Eating For Effect", will continue, very likely, indefinitely. My weight is nearly normalized. My initial target was 205 lbs. That has been achieved. I set a new target of 200 lbs, then195 lbs and the latter has recently been achieved. My new goal is 190 lbs. I am currently at 194.4 lbs.

Crucial to the success of the process is prayer. Additionally, I have had to make further reduction in breakfast intake and I have had to make sure that I have had plenty of exercise.

Reviewing the charts per weight and glucose control have also been very import.

Currently, the trends have been the best yet.

I am currently planning to enter a light weight lifting regimen, which may make it difficult to hold 190 lbs.

My intake has been heavily focused on foods like beans, tomatoes, zucchini, eggs, chicken and lean meats with most of the meat grilled or baked. Carbonated drinks have been minimal, flour products are still out and potatoes are also not eaten.

I have noticed, just recently, that small deviations in food intake have not seemed to hurt my glucose levels.

Two months ago those same deviations would have resulted in significant glucose spikes.

My morning readings have not been over one hundred for over 50 days. I have averaged 92 for the last three Months.

The same daily *routine* has been executed during the past (26) twenty six months. It is outlined later in this letter as well as previous letters.

For your review, I have brought charts reflecting weight reductions, blood pressure behavior & glucose behavioral charts. Unfortunately, I do not have Win Gluco Facts up running on our new system, but should be able to get that accomplished next week.

I have amassed almost 4000 glucose readings during the study period, and now believe that I am in control and only require one reading a day. I occasionally take 2- 4 readings to make sure things are working correctly.

Although I am not certain, I think the A1C results should be better than my last visit.

Data For Your Review,
      Glucose Charts
      Blood Pressure & Pulse Charts
      Weight Data Charts

All of these trends appear favorable

Here are other significant factors;

Intake	No Bread, potatoes, soft drinks (carbonated), or fatty foods. Hi Intake / Fresh Vegetables-Some Fruit Also Usually have Micro Eggs Moderate Intake (Roasted Chicken- Baked Fish) Nuts, Berries & Diet Ice cream nearly every day.
Frequency	Intake is Four Times A day (Includes a snack at around 8:00 PM)

Intake Size   small!

Glucose Reading Frequency   1 Times/ Day

Daily Routine (Preferred)

Morning	Noon	Dinner	Evening
Prayer	Glucose	Glucose	Glucose
Scales	Enter Data	Medicine	Blood Pressure
Blood Pressure	Intake Intake	Enter Data	
Glucose		Enter Data	*Prayer*
Medicine			
Intake			
Enter Data			
Evaluate Charts			

<u>My Wife & I have made serious changes in our lives</u>, and I think these will be permanent changes in thinking and behavior.

Perhaps the second most important change has been the investment of time to evaluate.

_____

Richard Phillips
PS

Two meters have been used with the majority of data per the Bayer Glucometer Elite.

<u>Your help along with Nurse 1 & Nurse 2 is sincerely appreciated.</u>

<u>I need to talk to you about glucose strips.</u>

Humbleness

Keep <u>Humble</u>. Remember, if you and I are "<u>In The Trenches</u>" fighting excess weight or glucose control, and or blood pressure or some other problem, <u>we are (likely) the bad guys that caused the problem in the first place.</u>

1. This is not always the case. Who was it that ate too much? Who was it that ate the wrong food? Who was it that ate at the wrong times? Who was it that skipped meals? *I know I am guilty*. In my case, it is answered prayer, and that has given me direction and resolve.

GOD is the one who should be thanked every day. *HE* is the one who cared enough to give us the proper direction in the first place. Keep <u>humble</u> and be thankful.

That attitude has been expressed as a desired attitude from the *CREATOR. JESUS* tells us about this in the New Testament, and we are told about this, thousands of years earlier, in the Old Testament.

Keep <u>humble</u> and maintain a thankful heart. *Don't take credit for success*. Keep <u>humble</u>, as you enjoy a healthier life.

And, with renewed success, hang on to the mighty ally, <u>Hope</u>!

Getting My/Your Life Back

Things happen. Often, they happen very gradually. Spring comes, plants turn green, some bloom, and some have leaves, then later the colors fade and then some become yellow, brown, or red, later losing their leaves. All of this takes time and happens gradually over a number of days, weeks, and months.

While some of us abused our bodies by eating for pleasure, some of the same people, and I am one, gradually lost physical abilities. In my case, it was only after I lost weight again, that I realized that I could now do things that I didn't realize I had lost.

Jogging across the back yard, feeling the wind in my face on a basketball court, feeling my knees lift higher, and simply feeling good, were some of the things that I got back! *"Staying The Course"*, following *"The Daily Routine"* including praying, staying <u>humble</u>, and being thankful, are all components of <u>getting my life back</u>, or having it given to me, once again.

81

You could say, <u>I got my life back.</u>

A Silent Killer

What people with diabetes must realize is that an uncontrolled system can do harm so <u>silently</u> and so slowly that by the time a person with diabetes realizes that a problem exists, it might be too late. Hearing, eyesight, heart failure, kidney failure, and other damage to the body can occur very slowly. High blood pressure often accompanies high glucose readings in people who have type 2 diabetes. With control, much of this damage can be avoided. Without control, increased risk of stroke and heart attack also exists.

Uncontrolled weight and uncontrolled blood pressure can cause many problems!

The problem I had was, <u>hear no evil, see no evil, and do no evil.</u> What that means (as mentioned earlier) is that by not knowing that a problem existed, then there was no problem, and everything seemed to be okay. I thought that if nothing was known to be wrong, then, nothing was wrong.

If I don't know that a problem exists, then surely, nothing is wrong. While I may think nothing is wrong, I could be setting myself up for major medical problems, including a problem that could be fatal.

The truth was, I did not want to know that there was a potential problem or a real problem. Not knowing allowed me to enjoy life. I would not have to make any changes, and living my life the way I was used to, including the pleasure of overeating, could continue.

Some of these potential problems could actually become fatal.

In a way, diabetes, uncontrolled, could become <u>a silent killer</u>.

The System

This is the term I use to describe my body's functioning components. As discussed earlier, glucose in the blood stream, blood pressure, and weight are what I refer to as *The System related dependent variables.* Sleep, exercise, stress, and solid-food & liquid intake are items that affect, *The System*. These are the independent variables. These are things such as, prayer, diet, exercise, sleep, stress, medicine, and other things which affect the system readings.

For example, if I eat too much food in my diet, it can and will affect the glucose reading, and in this example, it will cause my readings to be too high. Missing dosages may affect my readings. Stress affects my readings and this has been documented. Eating the wrong kind of food affects my glucose readings.

Following "*The Daily Routine*" helps me control my system to the extent that I can predict my glucose, weight, and blood pressure, fairly accurately.
Each system is unique. *No two systems are exactly alike*. *Every System Varies*. That is why it is essential to go through the entire process and not rely upon what has worked for someone else.

We can choose to go along for the ride, or we can try to control our system by driving where we want to go, and possibly have a much richer life. In many cases, it is up to us!

By following "The Daily Routine", we are choosing to try to understand our system(s) and then influence system behaviors in order to attempt to improve.

The Glucose System

My use of the term The Glucose System refers to glucose levels within the bloodstream, and the behavior of an individual's glucose levels (or readings). During the day, as discussed earlier, it is normal to see glucose levels change. They will rise and fall. Another term, variation, describes these changes. By studying the glucose readings, there are tendencies that are revealed, and are, likely, unique to each person.

What happens, during our daily life, influences the amount of glucose present in the bloodstream. It affects the variation or the changes relative to high and low readings. In my case, and probably most cases, when I need extra energy, I will usually see a higher level of glucose present. Normally, also in my case, the higher levels will drop back to normal, shortly after the need no longer exists.

After about 2000 readings, also previously discussed, it became apparent that <u>activities</u> such as public appearances were accompanied with higher than normal readings. The readings fell back to normal levels shortly after each public appearance. As professionals have stated repeatedly, stress can cause glucose readings to change. This was reinforced by studying activity records, and comparing them to glucose readings. Those records revealed that making public appearances, leading worship services, chairing local committees, and presenting music to audiences, generally elevated my glucose readings.

The <u>food</u> that I eat or <u>drink</u> and the type of food that I eat will also have effects upon my system. The key for me was learning to understand the effect eating food or drinking liquids had, and/or has, upon my <u>system.</u>

There were certain foods that I ate that had very little effect, while others had enormous impact. During my examination of my <u>glucose system</u>, I found those foods which worked well, and I found those foods which needed to be avoided.

<u>Exercise</u> also played an enormous role in controlling glucose readings. The simple act of walking or trotting had huge, positive effects upon my glucose levels.

Finally, <u>Prayer</u> has provided balance and has helped bring my <u>glucose system</u> back to normal levels. T<u>rying to handle problems over which I have no control has already been discussed.</u> I mention that because prayer plays a major role in stress management. Prayer makes a difference!

The importance of having a good spiritual condition <u>*(prayer)*</u> was, and is, essential to my journey, and <u>*prayer may be the single, most important component of all that I do.*</u>

The Controlled Glucose System

A <u>controlled glucose system</u> means that I can predict glucose levels, before I actually take the reading. It refers to the knowledge of past glucose readings or behavior, the knowledge of present glucose levels, and the ability to accurately predict my future glucose level. It also includes running levels with few surprises. If I average 100 but also vary by 100 points from one reading to the next, I do not have a controlled system. The variation is too extreme.

For example, I can accurately predict my glucose level and behavior and I have an understanding of where my system has been. I know that with the current medication, with the same solid and liquid intake (food), and on days with normal activities, I will average about 100 with the day starting at or below 100, and then rising about 10 points for lunch, then dropping below my starting point at the third meal (dinner), and slightly rising again at about 9:00 P.M.

For people with scientific or detail-oriented backgrounds, I want to see about an even number of readings above and below the nominal reading and I want to see readings fall within plus or minus 3 sigma. About 68% should fall within plus or minus 1 sigma, about 95% within plus or minus 2 sigma, and about 99.73% within plus or minus 3 sigma. If that happens, we can say the distribution is normal, hence, I have a controlled process. This is all technical stuff that is really not needed in order to have success with "<u>The Daily Routine</u>". It is, however good information for someone who wants to know.

To get the results that I and my wife have achieved, simply getting into a safe range, prescribed by our doctor, and then hitting the A1C targets and being able to predict and achieve good levels ahead of each meal time, means that we have achieved control.

There are those in the medical field who will dispute the ability to predict accurate levels, yet, we do it often.

That was not always the case.

Part of the difference between controlled and capable lies with the ability to accurately predict (controlled) vs. being able to accurately predict and achieve a good average and range that fall within the safe area.

The Capable Glucose System

The last paragraph above says the very same words.

Part of the difference between a <u>controlled system</u> and <u>capable system</u> lies within the ability to accurately predict (controlled) vs. being able to accurately predict and achieve a good average and range that falls within the safe area.

We are running predictable levels with minimal pre-meal variations. That means we have control. If the average or the range is too great, then we can say that we do not have a <u>capable system</u>. If I consistently predict readings that are too high, yet they are very predictable, I have a <u>controlled system</u>, but I do not have a <u>capable glucose system.</u>
Our goal needs to be to achieve <u>capability</u>.

To achieve <u>capability</u>, the first step is to control glucose readings. This could also apply to blood pressure or weight.

The second step is to get the average where the doctor wants it, and to keep the variation within the guidelines or target areas, set by you and your doctor.

The idea behind medicine, when systems fail to be capable or controlled, is to restore <u>capability</u>, which means that we will have levels where physicians want them to be, and we will know it in advance, and we will be able to predict the result.

Once that happens, the bombardment of numbers and readings can drop off radically and fall into an audit system, whereby a person checks every few days. As long as there are no surprises, then control has been achieved. As long as the readings are in the prescribed safe area, then <u>capability</u> has likely been achieved.

Your doctor can tell what your <u>system</u> is doing. He or she can prescribe the proper medication, and can also refer us to specific diets, but, it is up to us to build the resolve to do what we should, in order to get the best results for ourselves.

In many cases, our health is our responsibility.

Part of the goal here is to achieve <u>capability</u>. We want to operate within the target area outlined by the doctor and you. Along with <u>capability</u>, there is <u>Hope</u>!

Awareness

<u>Awareness</u> is another term used to describe the process of knowing what is happening, what has happened, or what will happen to our system. I can now predict my weight, glucose, and blood pressure.

I can be <u>aware</u> through the process of praying, reading, recording, analyzing, and then praying again.

In order to be <u>aware</u>, I not only have to Pray, read, record, and analyze, I must be willing to invest the time, daily.

By being <u>aware</u>, one can head off undesirable trends, while reinforcing those activities which help to reach goals and objectives.

Being aware is like being armed. <u>Awareness</u> provides one more building block for achievement.
Because I am aware, I have Hope.

Read It & Record It

Brooke

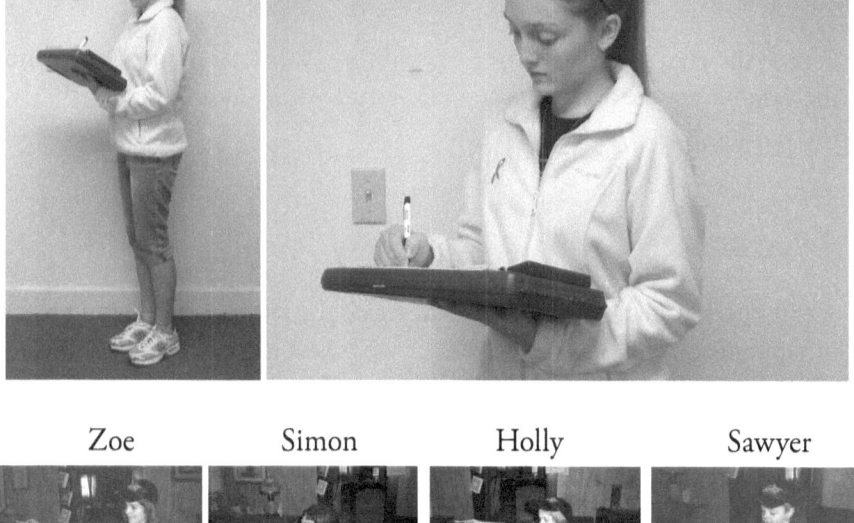

| Zoe | Simon | Holly | Sawyer |

When taking readings, it is important to take the attitude of *"Read It & Record it"*. Why? Over time, the importance of readings will become clearer. Looking too deeply into individual readings can often be a waste of time. It is the trend data that has the most significance.

The reason this is true is that there are always error margins to consider regarding individual readings. Trend data, however, is generally more accurate, providing the logger has good measuring instruments and is using them properly.

Taking a *"read it and record it"* attitude stresses the importance of doing just that. Take the reading, and write it down or enter it into your computer. After a while, it becomes routine. Finally, the logger simply does the job of logging as accurately as possible, and then, during the analysis, the report should generate a trend line and that is the main area to watch.

Elliot

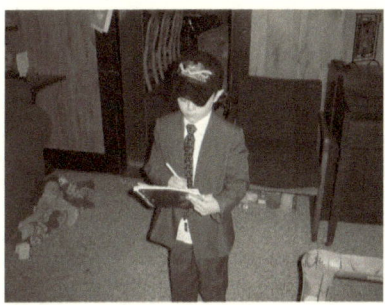

Here is the point. One person was alarmed at a <u>reading</u> of (systolic) 133 over 70 (diastolic) regarding blood pressure. The person was new at, "*<u>read it and record it</u>*".

After explaining that the blood pressure changes, almost minute by minute, and to report it to the doctor, this person continued to take spot checks and found that the overall trend looked good and that the 133, which was high, was not a representative number for her blood pressure.

Being alarmed translates into worry. Worry translates into stress. Stress is bad! Stress can not only affect blood pressure, but, it can also affect glucose readings. Simply get the facts and <u>record</u> that information and make sure to discuss with your doctor anything that looks unusual or problematic. Even if everything looks okay, give the information to the doctor! Show all the information to the doctor, so that the doctor can help you help yourself.

The other thing that needs to be said is that there are times when individual <u>readings</u> should be a concern. If they fall into the really high or really low area, they could be dangerous. In that case, contact your physician immediately, if that is the arrangement.

The danger zone can, and should be specified by your doctor. It is recommended that you have <u>a plan of action worked out with your</u>

doctor in advance to address cases where you may reach a danger zone. In other words, you might be able to do something like drink orange juice or take a glucose tablet if a glucose reading was way too low. There might be some special communication required depending upon your particular situation. If it is way too high, there might be some other prearranged action that you could take, or maybe communication with your doctor will be required.

Otherwise, simply "Read it and Record It."

Just Say No

When I first started "The Daily Routine", it was very difficult to break the habit of eating the wrong foods and eating too much. I learned that after praying, saying no really helped. I would Say NO mentally, and that changed a lot of my problems. What ultimately happened is that I was able, with some true effort, to avoid eating too much and to avoid eating the wrong foods.

If you think you are going to slip, remind yourself to *Just Say No!* Also, be aware that it gets easier, as time goes by.

We Don't Need As Much As We Think

When it comes to food, the truth is, I don't need as much as I think. If I intend to lose weight (and by now-I have), I want to do so safely. The volume of food I used to eat was easily (4) four times as much as I eat now. Also, the type of food that I eat is much higher quality.
If I eat red meat, it will be lean. I make certain to remove the vast majority of fat. I look at the meat that appears to be nearly fat free.
There are no fried foods. We simply grill, bake or broil. The next main concern is keeping portions small. Instead of a heaping, full plate of food, I eat much less.

When I eat (4) Four times a day, until the final meal at about 9:00 P.M., I know that I will get to eat again soon. As a result, I don't feel nearly as compelled to eat a huge portion or meal, because I know that it won't be long, before I get to eat again.

Another factor, which I mentioned earlier, is that I deliberately look for bland foods to eat. The desire to over eat or eat huge quantities of food that tastes poorly is simply gone.

The over powering urge, to overeat, ebbed primarily due to prayer. I cannot say that I spoke to _GOD_ and _HE_ said to do this or that. Yet, I believe crying out to _GOD_, out of desperation, resulted in answered prayer. From answered prayer, which is ongoing, my resolve has become part of "_The Daily Routine_". As each day, in the beginning, passed, I seemed to be less tempted to return to old habits.

Old Habits Are Easy To Resume

Old habits are easy to resume, but, I believe as long as I earnestly pray for "Staying The Course", and I continue to follow "_The Daily Routine_", I will never fall back into the same scenario of eating too much, not eating at the right times, and/or, skipping meals.

It is very unlikely that old food types will be permitted. Huge volumes of bread, fatty foods, and large volumes of carbonated liquids will very likely never again be a part of my regular diet.

If I am fortunate, my days will start and end with prayer.

Although we do not know how many days, hours, minutes, weeks or years that we have left, taking care of what has been given to us requires routine maintenance.
That takes us to "_The Daily Routine_".

The process of bringing this system to normalcy has been a long, slow, and deliberate process. I am grateful for what has been given to me. The truth is, I probably have been given a second chance.

I need to use that chance to do the right things, and make them count for something. _Resuming old habits should not be part of this process!_

If I do not pray, if I eat the wrong foods, get away from <u>read, record, and analyze it</u>, from experience, I know that <u>I can resume old habits</u> easily. This has happened several times, during the past nine years. It did not take long to realize a tighter waistline. What this means is simple. I need to stay with "<u>The Daily Routine</u>", because, I do not use good judgment without "<u>The Daily Routine</u>". Many people are probably not like me. They do use good judgment most of the time. Not me. <u>Old habits are easy to resume</u>.

Based on my experience, during the past (9) nine years, I have a great deal of <u>Hope</u>, because today I am doing very well, in spite of the time involved.

<u>Establishing Control Can Be A Painful Experience</u>

The change from old habits to new habits has been a painful experience. First, in order to <u>establish control</u>, I had to take about 125 glucose readings at each time of day (morning-noon-evening-night) or a total of 500 readings (@4 times a day for 125 each). That required about (4) four months time. The process of taking glucose readings, even though it is nearly painless, still was uncomfortable. The cost, hours of observation, the process necessary to collect the information, have all involved time and expense. I had to take at least four readings a day, on top of weighing daily, and that was costly for the price of glucose strips. I had to check blood pressure several times a day, and that required more patience. To reach the level of confidence to understand my particular system, I had to take enough readings to fairly and accurately predict what the reading would be, at specific times per day. As soon as a person can actually predict, within reason that is, weight, glucose levels, and blood pressure on a daily basis, *<u>control has been achieved</u>*. With control, I know what has happened, what is happening, and what will likely occur.

Maintaining Control

After control was achieved, I never wanted to go back to an uncontrolled status. I would not want to weigh too much, or to have my blood pressure too high or to have my glucose have wild swings and be too high.

The process of weighing daily may continue indefinitely, but, the process of taking glucose readings daily has already ended. As of the end of 2009, one glucose test, every few weeks, is now all that is required. The last A1C was 5.7. As of 2/17/06, control was first really established. With the A1C test, I can confirm glucose control. After about 2 years. I began testing once a day. The morning test, which was my worst time of day, became the bench mark, and my readings could be accurately predicted to run under 100. Now, in 2010, periodic sampling shows a continued controlled status. What that means is that even though I only test once over a several week period, I will pick a day at random, and make several tests at different times. This is an audit, and as long as I fall in the safe, predictable range, I keep the frequency at once every few weeks. These are pre-meal tests. (Read more on this subject later in the book, because there are revisions to the two week time frame.) Later data suggests more frequent checks should be made.

Eating For Effect

Now that control has been established and maintained, the discipline of _"Eating For Effect"_ is now a way of life. This process is now shared with both my wife and myself. If we see trends that indicate that we are slipping, and that does happen from time to time, we merely adjust our intake or, some other known variable, to re- acquire the goal. Weight can move up slightly, but, by taking daily readings, we can, and do, adjust our solid and liquid intake. I also step-up exercise. Glucose may move in the wrong direction. For us, that would be up. If it does, we can adjust our exercise, food intake, or some other known variable like stress, and watch the glucose fall back into the proper range. By "Eating For Effect", the reduced amount of necessary intake is, once again, fortified. Also, the proper food, and the necessity to eat proper food, is reinforced. This all revolves around _"Eating For Effect"_.

The truth is simple. We can identify foods that work well for us. We can eat the same foods day in and day out, with very little variation. We almost always have the same breakfast. We have a bowl of cereal with milk. (Sometimes I eat one or two hardboiled eggs). I also occasionally will beat eggs in a bowl and put them into the microwave. That works too. Scrambled or fried eggs are a rarity. Now, the cereal may vary, but I don't seek out the variation to satisfy a desire to eat something that tastes great or that tastes differently. I really try to avoid that scenario. (Watch the sugar content of the cereal) I target 4 grams or less.

"Eating For Effect" steers me to eat many of the same foods, day in and day out. There is more variation at lunch and dinner, but, the last meal of the day is usually the same food, every day. We generally have nuts, berries or diet ice cream or some variation of those foods.

"Eating For Effect" drives us to look for results rather than great taste. "Eating For Effect" results in eating a lot of the same foods, rather than high food variety. That really helps keep the numbers, on our report, where we want them.

Taking Charge

We can take charge of our life, or, we can let our life take charge of us. When I was eating too much, and/or eating the wrong things, I knew it. I knew that four hamburgers was too much to eat for one meal, and I knew that *fat-filled food* led to a *fat-filled body*. The pleasure of eating, in those days, outweighed, literally, the process of eating the right foods at the right times. I had to get to the point where, enough is enough! To use an appropriate pun, I simply got fed up! I was tired of losing the battles and the war!

With prayer as the prime mover, I was gradually able to take charge of my life.

Responding

<u>Responding</u> refers to the reaction that we have to information that has been read, recorded, and analyzed. We can accurately take readings. We can accurately record readings. We can accurately display readings. We can accurately analyze readings.

After going through all the trouble, including absorbing the time and cost of this process, we really need to <u>respond</u> by doing the right things that will bring good results.

There is something about seeing the information that often causes a person to adjust habits <u>(Respond)</u> in order to get better results.

We need to <u>respond</u>!

The Bank

My body is like a <u>bank</u>. In my case, <u>"the bank"</u> is where the body wants to conserve every ounce of energy that it takes in.

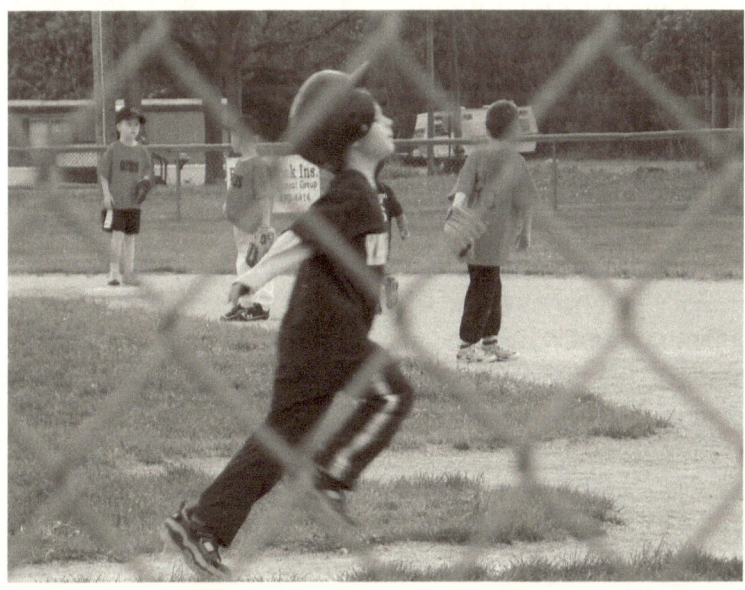

On the other hand, to make the withdrawal requires a lot of hard work. What this really boils down to is calories in vs. calories out. It's easy to put calories in. Why is it easy? That's simple. Food that tastes great is usually eaten in large quantities. Eat too much, and calories in will exceed calories out. End result is, a quick way to gain weight. This process that I am on is now going on ten years. On July 14th, 2015, it will be ten years that I have been going down this new path. Since I have had several periods where I stopped following the "The Daily Routine", I have solid evidence that, for me, it is a sure way to gain weight and lose control of a great life.

Now we are talking about the war again. This war of maintaining a healthy weight by eating right, eating the right number of times per day, eating at the same relative time of day and continuing to pray, read, record, and analyze, or otherwise follow "The Daily Routine" vs. not choosing to have a healthy life, should be a winnable war. And, I think it is winnable.

It's hard to take calories out. The problem has been described in earlier sections of the book. I get a great sensation of gratification from eating good tasting, bad for my body, food. It can be so overpowering that I can live my daily life with the expectation of "What do I get to eat next?" Notice the option. I get to choose. I can choose to follow a great path, or I can choose to stray from the path that has brought me success.

With that, comes the very slow deceiving and deceptive change in body mass. Once when I was slim and trim, I could do a lot of things. The deception was that eating good tasting; bad for our bodies' food did not cause any problem. From a size 38 waist to a size 58 waist took place over a number of years. There was no problem, so I thought, with "The Banks" conservative policy. We must store food for energy. It was no problem, because I did not slow down to consider what was really happening.

The problem actually was creating a danger to my health and well being.

One of the bad things about the Midwest is that we have 4 distinct seasons. For someone who needs to maintain an around the year high activity level, winter is a problem. What this really needs is a flexible personality who is willing to find winter activities that will result in high levels of productive exercise.

So what do I do? I try to keep informed. If I start to climb in weight, then, I should do something about it, before I get out of control. If I stop following "The Daily Routine", I can gain weight and not know it, until my pants are too small or too tight, and then I am behind, with a problem to solve.

The big difference has to be centered around following "The Daily Routine" through the winter! The key may lie with wintertime activities. Exercise!

Exercise

| Sawyer | Elliot | Blake |

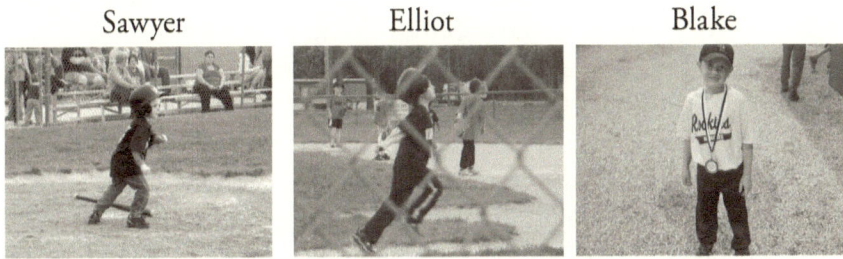

This is another area that I have more ideas about. In my younger days, I spent a considerable amount of time in the gym, lifting weights, playing handball, basketball, swimming, & hitting the speed bag.

One of the things that I learned was that, during weightlifting, I would work, until I was really exhausted. As I wore myself down, I would allow a day of rest for muscle rebuilding. Almost every week, after I began weightlifting, I noticed that I could lift more weight.

In essence, as I wore myself down, I seemed to come back stronger.

This same philosophy has been used, since I began recent regular exercise.

Today, June 22, 2010, it was nearly (90) ninety degrees. I played outdoor basketball for about 35 minutes, almost nonstop. I was soaking with sweat. Although it was nearly a continuous motion, I never worked hard enough to the point that I gasped for air. At the end of 35 minutes, I left the court, not because I was tired, but for safety. I was not sure how long I could work in that kind of heat, so I stopped, cooled off, and went back and mowed the yard with a rider.

When I was diagnosed with diabetes in 1998, I began to exercise regularly. I found something that I enjoyed, and it was something to which I looked forward (and still do). The bottom line regarding exercise is this: find something that you like to do. "*Staying The Course*" is much easier.

When I began, I weighed around 270 pounds, or maybe more. At the beginning, I could only exercise for about 5 minutes. Much like exercise in my younger years, as time went by, I seemed to gain more strength. It wasn't long, until I could continue for 10 minutes, then more and more, until I reached a point that I could continue for more than two hours. By that time, I had lost more weight.

As for the beginning of exercise in 1998, if I felt that I was getting almost too tired, I would drive home and sit down in the easy chair and cool down. I was fine, until I got out of the chair. Then, it was Tim Conway time. I felt 90 years old, and could only walk with very small steps, for a while.

At night, one or two elbows would ache. Sometimes it was one or two knees or some combination of elbows and/or knees. As a step to ease the discomfort, I would use a light wrap on the sore joint(s) and often would take an aspirin. Although exercise caused discomfort, something led me to believe that I needed to "*stay the course*", so, I continued to do this (6) six days a week.

Somewhere between (3) three and (6) six months, after I began to exercise regularly, I realized that I had no more aches and pains. Evening wraps were no longer necessary, and there was no need to take aspirin.

After sitting down and resting, when I got up to resume activities, there were no more stutter steps. I was also a little lighter.

Exercise played a large role in controlling diabetes, as well as managing weight. That was the reason that I started logging exercise and also ran correlation values against glucose and weight.

There is something else. Look up the term, "Neural Transmitter". I just did. Since 1998, the information on the internet has exploded. In 1998, my understanding was that neural transmitters were chemicals that attached themselves to the brain synapse and that they helped a person feel a sense of euphoria or well being. They also were natural pain killers. In addition, exercise played a large role in the balance and production of neural transmitters. Neural Transmitters enhanced communication, which meant that orders for the pancreas might be generated more effectively, if the neural transmitters were in a balanced state or were plentiful.

Today's information is much more complete, and, since I am not a medical professional, I will need to get information that is more detailed and built for a lay person, so to speak.

The theory that I developed was that trouble with diabetes might be linked to insufficient neural transmitters. By exercising regularly, with good intensity, I thought I could help my body perform its functions more effectively. Communication from the Hypothalamus to the pancreas might also be better.

The Hypothalamus acts much like a voltage regulator in an old car. The voltage regulator monitors the voltage going to the battery, until it is fully charged, and then redirects the voltage. The Hypothalamus monitors the blood stream and gives necessary orders to the pancreas to produce the proper amounts of insulin in order to hit target levels in the blood stream. It performs its function around the clock. Systematically putting good food in, at the proper volumes, and eating the same products, appears to significantly aid the functions of the body.

I look at the endocrine glands, and in this case, the Hypothalamus, as if it were a supervisor in a manufacturing plant. Some specialists look at it as if it were a thermostat. It senses, issues instructions, and maintains the areas for which it is responsible. Things like insulin are maintained to help the body function at optimum levels. Insulin and glucogon are two polypeptide hormones that control glucose levels in the blood stream. As an additional comment, there are other line supervisors, so to speak. Some other endocrine glands that are also involved in the regulation of insulin and glucagon are the pituitary, thyroid, adrenals, intestine and the pancreas.

One additional thing;
Hunger seems to be much less, when I have lots of <u>exercise. (Also controlled by the Hypothalumus)</u>

My documentation shows that <u>exercise</u> helps, and neural transmitters may be a byproduct of <u>exercise</u> and may play a large role in health.

It's 2014 now. With regard to <u>exercise</u> and perspiration, when I <u>exercise</u> outdoors (Basketball), I wear a cap, dark glasses, and normal <u>exercise</u> attire. I will almost always sweat profusely to the extent that even my cap will be saturated. When it dries, there is usually a white salt ring that will show. If it's leather, it may be damp for more than a day.

One must keep in mind that I have been doing this for a while and that it took time to safely build up to this level of activity. I seldom reach the point of being tired, but, I have added something new to my regimen lately.

I use 2.5# ankle weights on each ankle. When I first started doing this, this year, I noticed a slight knee joint discomfort. That has disappeared. I don't recommend doing this at all but, for me, it is a plus.
It works my body harder and may be playing a slight role in the new weight record lows that I have experienced. I hit <u>181.8 pounds</u> today (9/29/14) which is definitely the best I have reached during this (9) nine year journey.

I wear them all day, which means they will usually be on for a period of 12 to 16 hours. Most of the time, I am unaware that I have them on. I only do this three times a week. It's the same idea. Work the muscles and then give the muscles a chance to recover.

Additionally, when I wear the ankle weights and exercise outdoors, I do experience some fatigue. Some of the fatigue may be attributed to the fact that I have dropped from 205 pounds on April 29th, 2014 to 182.8 pounds on September 29th, 2014, so my reserves might be a little lower. After a few weeks, my endurance will probably be back to normal, which means when I leave the court, ankle weights or not, I will leave because it's a good idea to leave and not because I am tired. I would like to say that I am superman, but, that is not quite the case.

I am seeing some wonderful things with my glucose too. There are lots of readings in the 80's and 90's, which is what I look for when things are running in top form.

My Hope has been reinforced!

The professionals recommend exercise, and so do I.

TOD

TOD refers to the time of day, and the importance of taking medicine, and eating at the same time of day, every day. For example; when I take my morning medicine, I take it at approximately the same time of day, every day!

I take medicine before I eat. I usually have 15 minutes to a half hour, before I eat.
What usually happens is that I give my medicine a chance to start working, before I eat. My diabetes specialist encouraged taking the dose about 15 minutes, before I eat.

You may have to approach this differently, based upon your physician's directive(s).

Eating at the same <u>time of day</u>, morning, noon, evening, and in our case, 9:00 P.M., seems to gives the body a chance to regulate things. This appears to be a main, or important, factor for improving glucose control, and weight control. Every day, the call for insulin, digestive acids, and other things that relate to food intake & food processing, happens at nearly the same time. In effect, the system, or the program, may be expecting things to happen at a specific time.

The results of control have been great! With that in mind, doing things at the same time, within reason, may be part of better glucose control.

In effect, "<u>*The Daily Routine*</u>" is time-predictable for each day, with very small variations in <u>time-of-day</u>.

Self Indulgence

Achieving balance, to be redundant, has been a costly process. Medication that was really not necessary (under normal conditions), monitoring costs for glucose strips used to determine where my system was, and where it was heading, and where it eventually would be, has been costly.

<u>Self indulgence</u> has simply not been worth the price.
What is the price of <u>self indulgence</u>? In my case, Poor Health!

What's the price of over eating food for pleasure? What is the price of not being able to bend over to do a minor task? What is the price of not being able to climb a ladder? What is the price of carrying an extra 50 pounds or an extra 130 pounds all day long? What is the price of working my heart overtime to pump blood to a much larger than necessary body? What is the price of pumping blood that is much thicker? What is the price of working my heart overtime to digest a huge meal? (A meal that is two or three times larger than it should have been)

<u>Self Indulgence</u> is simply not worth the price of poor health.

That's Not All!

Consider the pocket book! Now, because I eat less, I have more cash to spend on things that can actually help me achieve or maintain a healthy weight.

Things like power tools, a tiller, router, bicycle, etc., etc., are now part of my equipment.
Self Indulgence is simply not worth the price of poor health.

As an added note, if you are fighting obesity, get two (5) five gallon containers, and fill them with water. That will be about (40) pounds each. Try walking with one or two of those containers full of water, and the effect will become clear, almost immediately. It is a heavy load and really puts an unnecessary strain on the body.

Again, I say, "Self Indulgence is simply not worth the price of poor health!"

Variety of Foods

In my opinion, needing lots of food variety is a myth. After 11 months of following "The Daily Routine", and taking about 1500 glucose readings, during the same period, I was able to discover foods that worked well with my diabetes, and foods that did not.
What I discovered is that eating those same foods resulted in good glucose numbers. Eating at the same time of day, gave me excellent results. For example, one or two micro-waved or hardboiled eggs for breakfast gave me good numbers at noon. A bowl of dry cereal with 2% milk and no sweetener gave me the same good results. Those cereals had to be 4 grams or less for sugar content. I identified foods at lunch, usually fresh fruit, vegetables, and light salads, that gave me good results at 5:00 P.M. Meals eaten at 5:00 P.M., that resulted in good results at 9:00 P.M., became part of my regular diet.

The main thing I learned was that lots of variety was not necessary. Most of my friends simply could not follow this process at the beginning. However, following "The Daily Routine" may change their minds.

If someone had told me on July 15, 2005 that I would not eat large amounts of food and that most of the time, I would eat the same food at each meal, I would not have believed them.

It is now 2010, nearly five years later, and every morning, with very few exceptions, I still eat either a bowl of milk and cereal, or I have one or two eggs that are hardboiled or a small omelet cooked in the microwave. This concept is also covered in the chapter called, "Eating For Effect".

The truth is, variety is not important for me. It is easy to say, after following this process, but in the beginning, I would not have even thought about eating the same food at the same time of day, nor would I have thought about eating four times a day.

Lots of Food Variety is Not Necessary, but HOPE is.

The Subconscious Mind

As I mentioned in the beginning, *I am not a medical professional* in any sense of the word, medical. What I am saying is what I believe. Whether or not science already has confirmed this theory or hypothesis, or not, is not known to me. What I do believe is that the subconscious mind records everything seen, heard, felt, or otherwise sensed. I also believe that the subconscious mind will help us achieve goals and objectives. I think that feeding visual data or images from taking readings to recording those same readings to analyzing those readings provides ammunition for the subconscious mind to help each person achieve goals and objectives.

I think that while I am sleeping and while I am awake, this wonderful tool is available to me and is working for me. As a result, when glucose behavior is recorded and analyzed, those things that need to happen in order to achieve a normal, or controlled, capable system, take place or are enhanced.

The subconscious mind knows where we have been, where we are going and where we need to go.

That, is the theory.

Following "_The Daily Routine_" really helps achieve high levels of performance.

Remember that prayer is the cornerstone of "_The Daily Routine_". The purpose of "The Daily Routine" is to provide a tool to achieve goals like weight, glucose and BP control. As a result, I think that the subconscious mind plays an important part of our success, not just in this application, but in all goal-oriented tasks.

The Journey

If someone had told me in 2005 that I would begin a new way of living, that I would purposely avoid good tasting foods, that I would eat (4) four times a day, and that I would achieve a normal or near normal weight level, and that I would live a much fuller life, I would have been very doubtful.

Part of the reason for the doubt is that I did not realize I was not living a full life. I had no idea what I had lost.

This journey is a journey of thanks. Thank you _LORD_ for this! I am not deserving, but I am ever so grateful. Thank YOU again and again.

Eating for pleasure, which still lingers, has almost vanished. "Eating for Effect", or following "_The Daily Routine_", has become my focus.

This is, truly, a wonderful journey, full of Hope.

Panning For Gold

The process of following "The Daily Routine" revealed that something was very valuable and I did not realize it. All I was trying to do was get my glucose under control and then my weight and then Blood Pressure. I was not thinking about the quality of life that was missing. But, in the beginning, I was worried about the possibility of having to take insulin.

It was only after I had made significant progress that I began to realize that I was regaining a much better life.

Finding that which is valuable is often difficult. It can be time consuming and rare!
In my search for value (gold), I have found that the pleasure of eating is a passing event (no pun intended).

The real value, or gold, lies in the time between meals, rather than during meals. So, with changed eating habits, by eating less, by eating more frequently, and by eating with less variety, I have found gold!

My gold is a higher quality of life. It (*a higher quality of life*) is a joy that lasts longer than the time it takes to eat a meal. It (*a higher quality of life*) is a joy that lasts longer than the time it takes to eat a meal. I have stated the idea twice for a reason. The gold was in front of me all the time. I just did not get it!

In my case, this realization has taken a long time to recognize. This did not happen overnight. Be Patient! There is Hope!

I have to emphasize that this process, this gold that I have discovered, is a gift. I take no credit for this. Once again, one day a prayer was made, and the next day, a change began.

Everything that I am doing now did not begin on July 15th, 2005. I know I have said this before. However, much of what I am doing now did begin on that date. As time went by, it became clearer that other steps were needed that would bring more benefit to me. Some items that I am currently monitoring were not recognized as important in the beginning. Now, they are routinely noted. Some of these things may cease to be monitored, after I have attained the optimum levels.

I have found *gold*, and, I am thankful!

Passing Moments

This is something that I did not think about, until I followed "The Daily Routine".
This is an area that really needs to be read more than once. There are some key phrases that helps truly describe this process. Here we go!

Moments are just that. They are here and then, they are gone. Their duration is momentary, or only for minutes, seconds, or parts of seconds. In any event, moments are quick. *Some are memorable, while others pass into the sunset of time*, never to be recalled.

Our life is momentary. We are here, then, we are gone. In the sands of time, our life on this planet is like a grain of sand on the beach of eternity. It sounds poetic, yet, when I think about immortality vs. our life time, I think it is a good analogy. A grain of sand on a beach is minute in size and content, compared to all the grains of sand that make up the beach.

Realizing that we are here for only a short time, the real questions are;

How important are our moments?

Are we spending our moments wisely?

How important are the moments we spend eating?

How long will those moments last?

Do we wish to accumulate a mass of moments that are valuable to us, centered on eating food?

For me, these questions help put things into perspective.

Do we wish to accumulate moments in other ways, like feeling the wind in our faces, as we move from place to place, enjoying the ability to once again jog, run, or trot a few feet here and there?

Do we get joy from trying on a new set of clothes? This might be a set of clothes that we could not wear a few months ago, because we were over weight?

If we don't spend our time, or <u>moments</u>, eating good tasting, fatty, large plates of food with seconds or thirds, how will we survive? How will we pass our time on this planet?

It is up to us to select our <u>moments</u>, which become *Passing Moments*.

It is my opinion that there is a difference between living life and existing. There is a difference between being a spectator and living an active life. There is no question that at 185 pounds I can live life rather than be a spectator. With living life comes active enjoyment. With being a spectator comes passive enjoyment. The question being, how do we want to live our lives?

We are all different. With me, my choice is to be actively enjoying life. I want to live life to the fullest. I want those <u>moments that pass</u> to be lived fully.
Enter "<u>The Daily Routine</u>".

Training Wheels

On two occasions, during this journey, two medications were reduced, over time, to zero. I was taking (4) four pills a day for one of two medications. Both of these medications were for control of diabetes. One of those medications (4 pills/day) is still at zero. It is gone. <u>As mentioned before, this can be done only with the consent of the physician.</u>

After a brief time, the glucose numbers began to creep up. I ultimately ended up taking only one pill for control instead of 5 pills a day.

Anticipation is an important part of the process. Anticipation can also be a negative force. If I anticipate trouble, then stress may enter the picture. Stress is a known variable, and can cause people with type 2 diabetes to have elevated glucose readings. In my case, this has been thoroughly documented.

Sometimes, taking a small amount of medication can put our minds at ease, and it is possible that medication may actually not be needed.

I refer to that situation as <u>training wheels</u>. Similar to learning to ride a two wheel bike, <u>training wheels</u> provides security, until the bike can be safely ridden without <u>training wheels</u>.

The bottom line is this. If I am working with my doctor and want to reduce my medication, but worry about the result, instead of simply reading, recording, and analyzing information, glucose readings may be actually higher due to the anticipation of glucose control problems. If that is the case, then a small amount of medicine may be required as a result of stress. I refer to that as <u>training wheels.</u>

Prayer has helped me eliminate worry, and as a result, I have been able to get to the minimum required dosage of medication. Therefore, <u>training wheels</u> don't apply here, but, they could have.

Jacob & Esau:

Esau would do anything, such as sell his birthright, for a good dish of food! Not only would he do it, he did it! He had some justification. He was hungry! He probably was not addicted to food, but was just famished from lack of eating. I have a feeling that I could have identified with the feeling Esau had. My problem was that I had that feeling of being famished nearly every day, even though I had eaten plenty of food. So addicted to food was I, yes, I did use the term addiction, that it was one of the central things on my mind for years.

Take Nothing For Granted

The fact that I know that I feel good, the fact that I know I am better physically, and the fact that I know that my endurance level is better and has increased significantly, does not, in any way, mean that I know that I am going to live longer.

It means to me that I am going to, physically speaking, enjoy my life better. If my physical condition is better, then I am going to be better emotionally. If I am better emotionally, then my glucose will run better. I think it will also help me keep a very thankful attitude, when I am speaking to our *CREATOR.*

The primary thought here, is that I must remain humble. A better life by following a wonderful path is no assurance that I will still be here an hour from now. It is, however, a better way for me to be here for that hour. I am very grateful.

Therefore, don't approach this process with the idea of taking anything for granted. Yet, if you are able, you can have confidence that a higher quality of life is there for the taking, if you choose to take it. There is Hope!

The Daily Log (Form)also see page 28

The Daily Log has, over time, gone through a number of revisions. Ours is a custom built, computerized spread sheet. We use the log to record data and then analyze information to adjust behavior early, in case we head in a wrong direction. Prayer was not added to the list, until almost a year and a half, after beginning "*The Daily Routine*." Even though prayer was, and is, a large part of the process, and was a huge part and was the first thing I did in the very beginning, it was not listed on the log, until December 17, 2006.

The component of prayer should have been the first step on the log sheet. Now, it is.

In The Beginning, my <u>Daily Routine</u> should have been as follows:

<u>Morning</u>	<u>Noon</u>	<u>Dinner</u>	<u>Night</u>
Prayer	Prayer	Prayer	Prayer
Scale-Weight	Glucose	Glucose	Glucose
Glucose	Systolic	Medicine	Intake
Systolic	Diastolic	Intake Food	
Diastolic	Pulse		
Pulse	Intake Food		
Medicine			
Exercise			
Citrus Intake			
Sleep			
Stress			
Coffee			
Record The Data			
Evaluate the			
Record			
Intake Food			
Charts	Charts	Charts	Charts

Prayer

<u>In reality, today's Daily routine-2014</u>

Prayer
Rest Room-Empty Bladder &/Or Colon
Scale-Weight
Medicine
Glucose (As Needed)
Read
Record

<u>Then record from the previous day:</u>
Exercise

111

Sleep
Stress
Solid Intake
Liquid Intake
Coffee
Ankle Weights
Analyze- the Record (Log)
Evaluate The Chart(s)

Prayer

Daily Log

Date										
Prayer										
Weight										
Systolic										
Diastolic										
Pulse										
GL Accessibility										
GL Speed										
GL Definition										
Glucose/Morning										
Exercise										
Sleep										
Stress										
Coffee/										
Intake/S										
Intake/L										
Medicine										

Breaking The Routine-The Planned Reward

Periodic <u>breaks from the routine</u>, after and during successes, are encouraged. The old saying;*"All work and no play is not good"*, applies here. Occasionally, I will deliberately reward myself with a meal that is simply eaten for pleasure. I still limit the food to low sugar content, but I still cheat by eating foods that otherwise are not good for me. Pizzas, a hamburger, spare ribs or some other food that is really bad will be eaten. The logging continues and disturbances are noted. Otherwise, I simply have a meal that is one that I really enjoy. I would not recommend this during the first 45 days. After success has been realized, I think it is a very good option, as long as one returns to the process immediately following this reward for doing well on "The Daily Routine".

Additionally, if I see trends that are unfavorable, I do not reward myself with a break in the routine. It has to be earned. This is one more thing that can act as a motivator. Consider the fact that I know that the time from one meal to the next is not very long. It follows that if I hit benchmarks, records, or goals and/or if I have sustained a really great level of control, and if I have demonstrated discipline, then a reward is justified and enjoyable, and encouraged. As such, I simply take a break, for one meal! This is comparable to taking a mini break and recharging my batteries.

However, it must be earned. Throughout this process, Hope remains a constant companion.

Computerized Charts In Excel

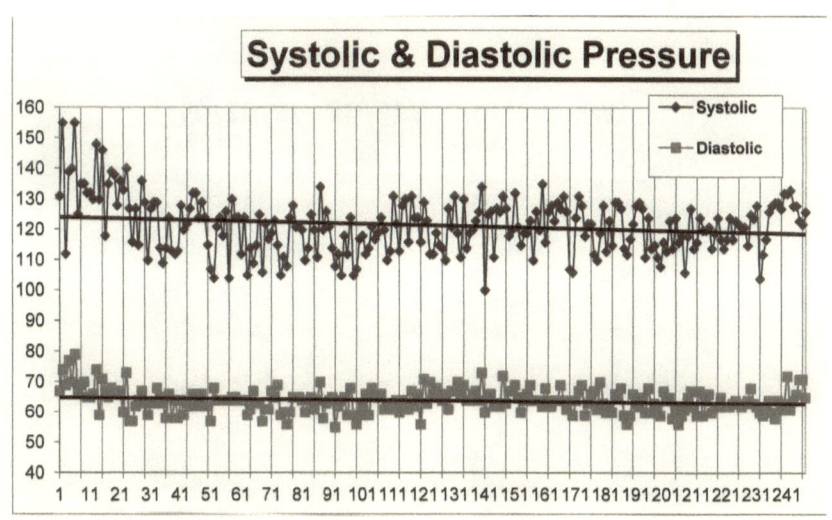

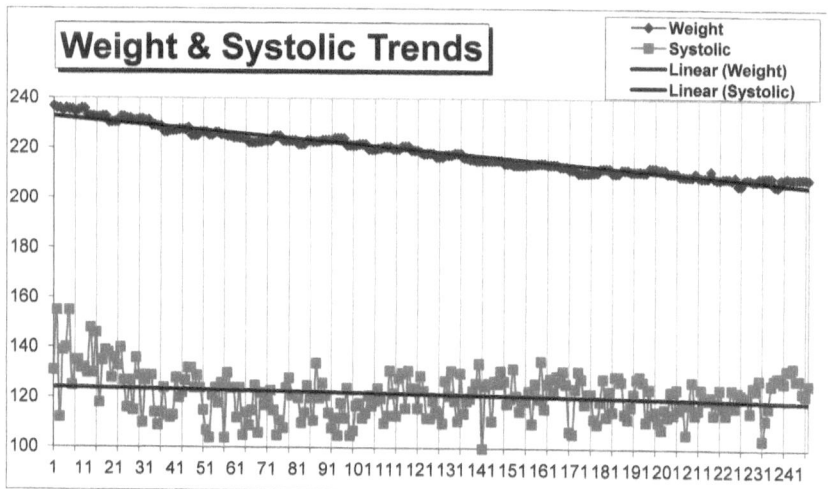

The First 4 ½ Months

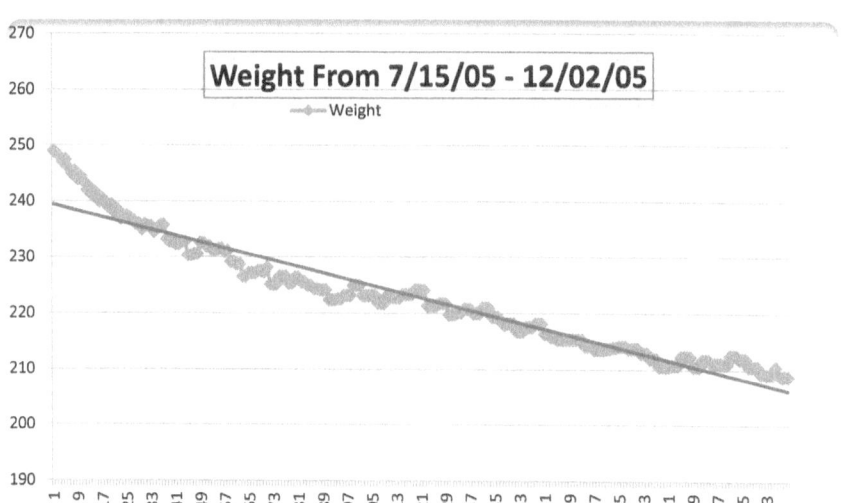

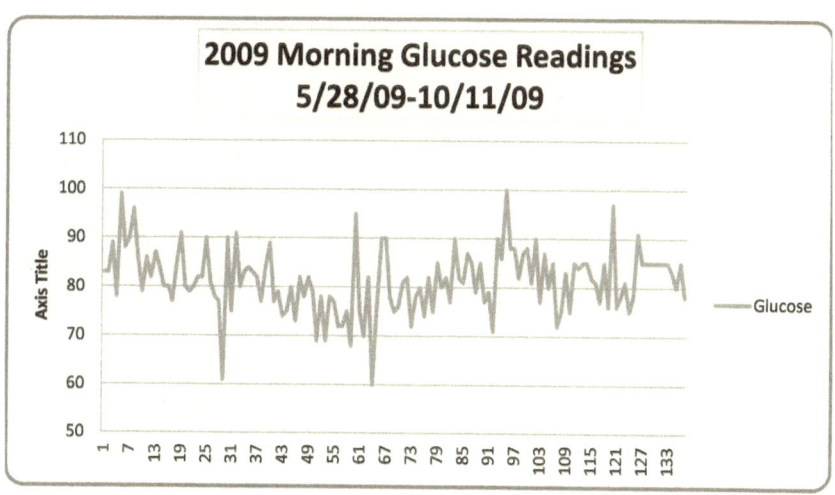

2009 Morning Glucose Readings 5/28/09-10/11/09

Axis Title

Glucose

Some Monitored Items from 2005

Early in 2005, these
are the items that were
<u>monitored</u>

Variables

	Later	More Recently
Weight	Weight Loss	Prayer
Systolic	Weight	Temperature
Diastolic	Systolic	Cum Weight Loss
Pulse	Diastolic	Weight
Glucose	Pulse	Systolic
Exercise	Glucose	Diastolic
	Exercise	Pulse
	Sleep	GL Accessibility
	Stress	GL Speed
	Coffee	GL Definition
	Intake	Glucose/Morning
		Exercise
		Ankle Weights

Sleep
Stress
Coffee/
Intake/S
Intake/L

Medicine

Achieving Balance

Spiritual   Mental   Physical   Perception

As of December 15th, 2010, it has been about (5) five and a half years, since I began this new path. I can say, "Thank you Lord for this."

Summary

Throughout this story, a central theme of Hope has been present.

The illustration of my many failures caused by doing things my way, until something new happened, is a small part of the story. It's the something new that happened that is the story. Something new happened after a desperate prayer was made on July 14th, 2005. On July 15th, 2005 a new direction emerged. It's the something new, "The Daily Routine", the new direction, that gave me Hope, and throughout this journey, Hope has been the mainstay and my almost constant companion.

It's important for me to say the credit for the change is not mine. I am just the lucky recipient of the change. When you look at it from the sidelines, what you see is a person who was in real trouble that needed help. My prayer was just that. It was a sincere, strong, profound plea for help. And, I fortunately received a positive response, because the answer gave me a new direction.

One day I was going in the wrong way, the next day I started on a new road that has brought me so much joy and Hope. At that time, for the first time in years and years, there was some victory.

After laying out the background of my story, we finally get to the new path that I walked. This new route, called "The Daily Routine", has been a journey that is still ongoing. On this journey, to this day, there is much Hope!

None of this could have happened without answered prayer.

As I follow "The Daily Routine", a comparable philosophy with regard to knowing where you stand that includes Read, Record, and Analyze could be similar to baseball or perhaps bowling. They each involve Effort, Preparation, Performance, and Feedback. Both endeavors are loaded with statistics, and, they each include Hope. A lot of Hope!

Baseball & Staying The Course

When the batter steps up to the plate, he or she never knows what will happen. All he/she knows is that the ball is going to be delivered, and, he/she needs to be ready to hit the ball out of the park. It may be a fast pitch, a slow pitch, a slider, a sinker, a curve, inside, or outside, etc., etc.,. The main thing is, be prepared. Do the work. Get used to looking for the ball. Anticipate, with reasonableness, that something good will happen. Then, take your swing.
Professionals spend days, weeks, months, and years preparing. Preparation is one key to success.
In my case, getting prepared for success is following "The Daily Routine". Praying is the first step. Stepping up to the plate is getting ready to follow the new path.

The mindset could be like this;

We never know what we will get when the day begins. All we know is that we need to be prepared, do the work, and then see what happens. Sometimes, what happens is a very great thing. Maybe, a home run will be hit, that is, we will see a significant weight loss. Maybe the batter will strike out, or nothing will happen. Who knows? The main thing is, play the game. Get in the game, step up to the plate, and then, when the time is right, take your swing.
It may help if the mindset of this new direction is based upon feedback. When you take your swing, do you know if you have hit a homer? Do you know if you struck out or hit a foul ball? Do you have information which will motivate you to step into the box the next time? Does what

you are doing help you to take the next step? Are you being encouraged or discouraged? Are you of one mind? (Are you committed?)

Now consider this: suppose you stepped up to the plate and each time you swung, you hit a home run. How exciting would that be? Day after day, always the same result. Month after month and year after year, the result would always be the same. Now suppose on the other hand, you always struck out. You never hit the ball and you never got on base. In either case, motivation to perform or get better simply would not exist. If we know the outcome before we try, why try? Are we getting better? Probably not. Are we getting worse? I have no idea.

We know that honest feedback is important and necessary, and in real life, that's the way the game is played. It's played with reliable feedback

Now, back to our process: At the beginning of the day, with the current game, "The Daily Routine", you never know what you are going to get. You prepare, work, and practice. Then you step up to the plate and give it everything you have. One thing is for certain. You will know almost immediately how you did or are doing. There is the real motivator. Success is a great motivator and if you do get a hit, or home run, there is no guess work on how well you did or did not do.

If you decide to follow "The Daily Routine", then consider our comparison to baseball.

The idea here is to follow the process and be sure to have feedback. Feedback is information that gives us an idea of how well we did.

Now, consider this,

Bowling

When a person throws the ball down the lane, they expect to see a good result. One usually hopes that all the pins will fall, but most importantly, you see the score or the pins that are down and those that are left, in the event that you did not make a strike.

119

The strength of this process is simply pointing out the important value of monitoring. You know the score. You are in position to do something about the score. You do not have surprises.

Oh, only knocking down one pin may surprise you alright, but you know that you only knocked down one pin and you can make an adjustment to compensate on your next attempt.

On the other hand, suppose you throw the ball down the lane. At the last second the pin setter raises the pins and then the ball sails through and knocks down-----nothing. Then the pins come down and reset. Your effort was for nothing.

Now suppose you throw the ball down the lane, and regardless where it strikes, you knock down all the pins.

You have the same result. You do not see the true value of your efforts.

If you are on a diet and the scales read random numbers or always read the same, you do not see the result from your efforts. Hence, there is no reward or motivation.

Seeing positive results provides fuel to continue to move in a positive direction.

Feedback, good or bad, is essential. Positive feedback really helps one move forward. It boils down to knowing. Knowing the truth allows us to evaluate our position and gives us information that we need in order to address the truth. The thing is this. If we do not know that a problem exists, then how can we do anything to correct the problem?

2014

In 2014, (9) nine years have passed since I began this new path. There is a major change in "The Daily Routine". First of all, every time I have gotten away from "The Daily Routine", regardless of the fact that the routine today is slightly different than it was a few years ago, I have had trouble managing my weight and my glucose control. Today, instead of taking glucose readings several times a day, the frequency is much less.

The fact is, I check my glucose in spurts. Usually, every few days is adequate. Often, I will run pre-meal checks at different meal times. The charts have a comment insert area that allows me to specify time of day and any pertinent information regarding that individual reading. For historical purposes, this has proven to be very valuable.

Before I step on the scale, I will always empty my bladder, and if convenient, my colon. In essence, I do those things, within reason, that will help me see the lightest weight. This relates back to motivation. The lighter I weigh, the more likely I am to "Stay The Course."

"The Daily Routine-2014"

Morning
Prayer
    1: Read

Bladder Empty/Colon
Scale
Glucose
Systolic
Diastolic
Pulse
Medicine-take

2: Record The Data
    & Other Variables such as
    Food Intake
    Sleep
    Stress
    Coffee Intake
    Liquids Intake
    Intake Food
    Charts

Note....... The log is filled out in the morning and items like food intake, liquids, and stress, are logged from the previous day's activities.

When I start my day, the first thing that should happen is to offer a prayer of thanks. Thanks for being able to wake up. Thanks for being able to get up. Thanks for the day. This part of the process was true in the beginning, even though it was not recorded, and it is true today. I need to talk with GOD, not just about this, "The Daily Routine", but about all matters of importance. Somehow, my balance or effectiveness as a human being is all related to starting the day, talking to GOD.
I have to confess, that this does not always happen. "The Daily Routine" helps, because at the very top of the routine is the word "Prayer". If I have not taken time, when I first wake up, then, there is a mental shirt sleeve tug to remind me of what I should have already done. Then, my day can be what it should be.

The next thing I do is head for the rest room. There, I do what most people need to do in the morning, and that is simply empty my bladder. Then, I to go to the scale in the same flat location and then turn it on. I step on the scale and get a digital readout. I make a mental note of that reading and then later, the information is put into the computer. I can also write the info on a piece of paper, if a computer is not available. Next, I no longer have to take glucose readings every day. When I do I take my glucose reading, it is recorded in the computer. As of 2014, I take readings every few days. Once in a while, I have a day where I will take several readings. If everything looks good, then I resume with the same frequency of once every few days. The readings are recorded, once again, on the computer. As of 2014, I do not feel comfortable waiting for 2 or more weeks to make a glucose test. That is a long time. I want to make sure that if there is a change in behavior, that I catch it early.

Let me expound on this for a minute. Earlier this year, I had a jump in my A1C. Last year, I had two significant injuries. Those events can cause a rise in glucose levels, all by themselves. There was, however, an additional element that also may cause glucose levels to rise or may cause other readings, renal related, to go sour. My A1C was 7.5, which is very high for me. Because both injuries involved a considerable amount of pain, and I do not take pain medication, generally speaking, I took Ibuprofen for an extended period of time. This could have been the contributing factor to affect some readings in a bad way. Once this was identified, (I had already stopped taking Ibuprofen for a few days), I was directed to stop taking that medication. Within a matter of weeks, my readings fell back into safe levels and the A1C dropped to 6.5. That is not bad, but still above my target. The doctor was happy, and I was glad for the improvement. The reason for mentioning this is that periodic glucose checks should reveal a higher than normal glucose level in situations like this, and they did. The rise in the A1C was predicted by me and shared with the doctor, and I decided that waiting for two or more weeks to check my glucose was not a good idea, so today I check every few days, as described, and then usually pick a day to run 4 tests to make sure that, during the day, I am running in a safe mode, so to speak. I have to say that "The Daily Routine" has been a learning process and has truly helped me understand my system.

Finally, blood pressure readings are taken and the same process ensues. Since weight control is my most challenging goal, I still take readings in the morning, before eating, and, I still record that information. (Every Day)
If I am not satisfied with that reading, I will often take it again at noon or later in the day, anticipating a loss of weight through higher activity levels. If the weight is lower at any time of the day, it's the weight that gets recorded. I also place a note described as a comment in Excel.

Let me give you an example. One day recently, following a day where I drank a lot of orange juice and water, I weighed 189 pounds in the morning. That, I did not like. I noted the log and took two readings later in the same day. I got some exercise by pushing our mower on a warm day hoping it would take some weight off. The second reading was 187.4 pounds and the last reading was 187.0 pounds. I really wanted to see 186 point something, but still was glad to see the 187.0 reading. The reading in the log showed 187.0, but in the comment section I noted 189.0 indicating that I really needed to watch the excessive liquid intake. Both conditions provided incentive to do more to keep the weight under control and it made the days' effort gratifying. As I said, the excessive liquid that I drank was orange juice. It tastes great. I had two full glasses of it and then had some water later. I really filled up on liquids that day and it showed on the scales the next morning. If I had not drunk the orange juice, I know I would not have drunk as much liquid, because I would not have been as thirsty. This gets back to lack of moderation. That is just me.

Regarding weight control and reaching new low levels of weight, a new strategy has emerged. About two years ago, I eliminated the riding mower. Since then, all mowing has been performed with a walk behind power mower. What I've realized, is that there is a significant amount of weight loss during the mowing activity, when I have to push a mower. In order to see lower numbers, I have decided to weigh myself again following the mowing activity. This year I have seen great results in one or two pounds of lost weight. This is particularly true during days that are hot. The lower number is entered into the computer and serves to provide motivation toward goal achievement. Many of the record lows, for weight management this year, have been achieved using this process. Currently the record low is 181.8 pounds.

Not only that, but the general average weight is now running at an all time low. This is true for a matter of weeks, and the current trend looks great. The thing is, due to the fact that I am running lighter, and want to stay that way, I think more intently about what I am eating, and simply dial down the volume as well as do a better job of choosing proper foods to eat. It all works hand in hand, and is fortified by prayer. As I am entering this information, at 11:30 p.m., I realize that I still have on 5 pounds of ankle weights that I have worn the entire day. That is remarkable and only serves to show that I am living a higher quality of life and enjoying it without even knowing that my body has worked a little harder during the day, and will likely get stronger over time by wearing these ankle weights.

Back to "The Daily Routine". Now that the information has been collected and recorded, I still analyze the information and look for trends. Trend data is provided in the chart section of my spreadsheet. I have created a chart that reflects the recorded information. Then I have a computer generated trend line that allows me to confirm the over-all direction, so that I can see progress or trouble. Is my weight gradually moving upward, going downward, or staying the same? The identical process occurs with blood pressure readings, when I take them. I do not take them every day at this time. (I can also see the numbers moving up or down, but the trend line is a great tool to ensure accuracy and control.)

Once all the information is recorded, I also record several other items such as, the amount of sleep I got the night before, and how much food I ate. There are other things that I consider important elements, which may affect glucose or weight readings, including stress, medication, coffee intake, etc., etc.,.

The idea behind "*The Daily Routine*" remains the same. One is that by reading, recording, and charting data, I am somewhat detached from the process. It seems to be a little less personal and it seems to be easier to be objective.
Two is that I am putting information into my brain, which allows me to be aware of what is happening. It is just possible, that with this information, the subconscious mind may be at work helping me achieve my goals. (This is probably a huge understatement). Many functions take place, and I am probably unaware of most of those activities, most of the time. It is possible that this process has helped me build resolve, or determination, and it may have also helped with actual biological functions to aid in weight reduction, blood pressure management, stress, and glucose control. This is hypothetical, but the fact remains that my system currently needs less assistance. My brain is still seeing more data and remarkable stability is being realized. In effect, I am doing my own advertisement (on myself), and, it seems to be working.

It has been 9 years since the beginning of this new direction. Today, I am at an all time low regarding my weight. It's August 20th, 2014. The record is 184.8 and a few days later, (8/26/14), I am 186.2. Am I going to worry about the increased weight? No! Am I going to put forth a little more effort to see the lower weight levels again? Yes! A few days have passed and a new record of 182.8 (9/24/14) has been achieved. Hooray!

I am now reaching a level where I expect the weight trend line to flatten, because I am at or close to my normal weight. This is truly a gift. Glucose readings are running in the 80's and 90's in the morning with very few exceptions.

The overall trend is still at an all time low.   Since adopting "The Daily Routine", I am living with HOPE.

I am blessed!

Improved Blood Pressure

As of July, 23rd, 2014, my doctor recommended cutting my medicine for blood pressure in half. What a blessing. I will have to monitor it and keep the doctor informed, but one thing is for sure, I do not need as much medication as I was taking.

This is one more benefit from the lower weight level that I am currently enjoying.

Losing Weight

Dropping weight will likely happen in spurts. In My case, I will sit on an area of weight for a while, like several days or a few weeks, and then suddenly drop one or more pounds. When that happens, I will take extra steps to help the downward trend, like back off on flour products like bread, go toward liquid foods more and keep fat intake low. Usually, I will step up the vegetables and fresh fruits and make a conscious effort to keep the meal sizes small. I stay with the 4 small meals a day plan, but pay more attention to what I am doing to make sure I give myself an advantage to hit a new low.

Usually, during the hotter time of the year, l will step up the outdoor exercise and then make a weight check after I have had a good workout. Things like mowing the yard and outdoor basketball really help me to hit the new lows. Another thing I do is make a bladder and colon check, before I step on the scales. If I can relieve myself of the fluids and solids, that will help too. This has to be done within reason. That is to say, if I do not feel the urge to go, I simply do not make the attempt.

It is during the warmer time of year that I will usually hit my low weight goal.

It is the colder time of year that I continue to struggle.

At the time that I make this particular entry, August 18th, 2014, my weight is at 187 pounds. The actual numbers read were 187.8. Using positive thinking as fuel for achievement, I claim 187 pounds, although in fact it is 187.8. The goal is to claim victory and focus on what got me there.

Remember the importance of being humble. It is sort of like walking softly and carrying a big stick. The walking softly is going about the business of losing weight and not bragging about it. The big stick is prayer and following "The Daily Routine" which emphasizes the importance of praying, collecting information, reading, recording, and analyzing information.

This achievement has been based upon prayer, which is part of the focus on "The Daily Routine". From April 29th, 2014 through September 29th, 2014, there is a remarkable chart of my controlled weight loss. That chart is available so that you can see, even after all these years, the benefit of "The Daily Routine". I will insert the chart so that you can actually see the results. The new low is 181.8 pounds.

Throughout this process, there has been encouragement and Hope.

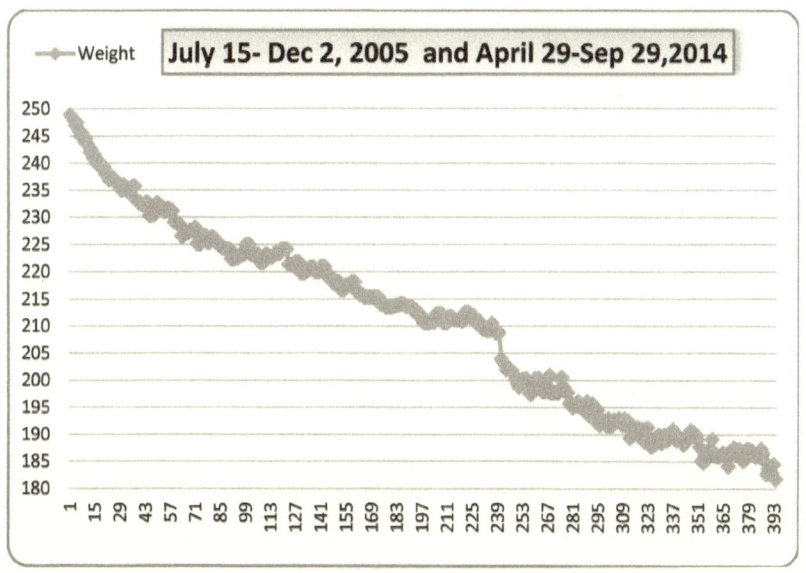

The above chart goes back to the very first day of "The Daily Routine". The first part of the chart extends from July 15th, 2005 through December 2, 2005. That is nearly (5) five months. It runs from point 1 through point 240. There are multiple readings on some days during the first period.

During the first period, I lost about 41 pounds and maintained that weight loss, with minor variations, for the next several years. I actually got below 190 at one point, but just barely, and never sustained that lower level.

The second part of the chart extends from point 241 through Point 393 and that is a (5) five month period in 2014. It takes me down to a record level in the 185 pound range. This is where I belong.

Over the years, I came close to this level, but never quite achieved it, until recently. A new strategy was initiated in 2014, which is part of the learning process of "The Daily Routine". It worked. It is described a little earlier in the section.

The data in the last chart is included in the chart above. It depicts the most recent activity and reflects the drop to my normal weight. Finally, I have reached the weight level that is optimum for me!

This is a blessing for which I am most grateful.

There is something else that needs to be emphasized here. In almost every case where there has been a focus on weight reduction, there has been a commensurate improvement in glucose control.

The following chart shows a weight gain in 2007, caused by not following "The Daily Routine" properly. When the weight went up, shortly afterward, so did the glucose numbers.

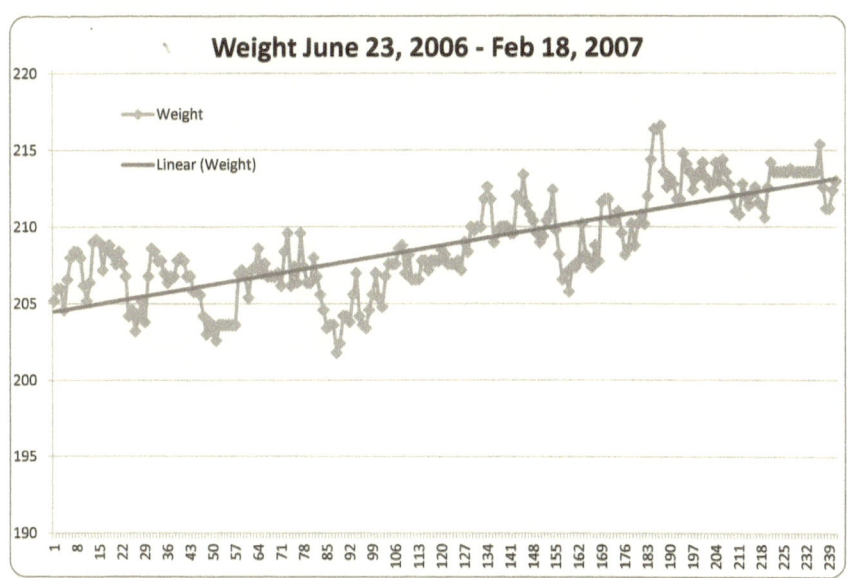

Weight June 23, 2006 - Feb 18, 2007

As stated before, during the nine plus years that I have followed this new path, there have been some lax periods. Actually, looking at the chart, June, July, and August and into September looked fairly good, but after about 90 days into this chart, there was a significant change and weight got out of control. Right after that happened, the following chart shows a loss of control with glucose.

During my experience with "The Daily Routine", there has always appeared to be a strong correlation between good weight control and good glucose control. My doctor told me that as well, and that point is documented in one of the enclosed letters, during which I recounted his advice.

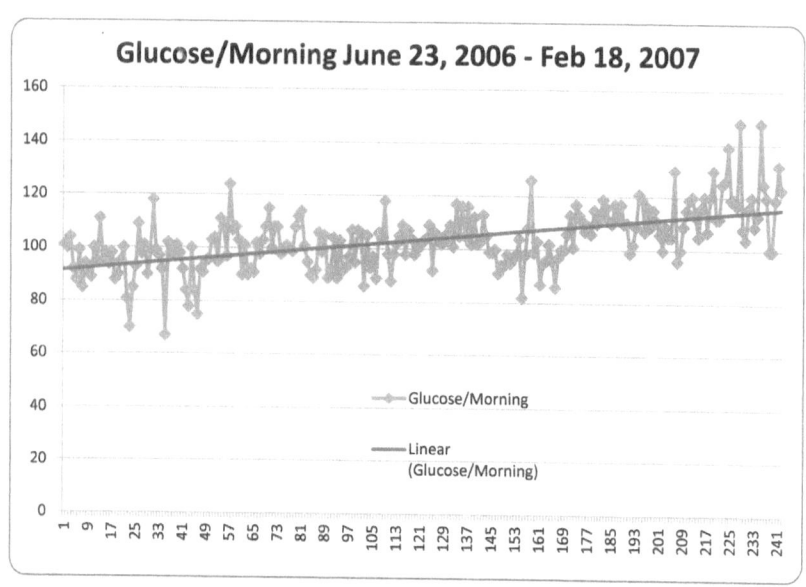

The following two charts which are reporting weight and glucose behavior in 2007 show the same behavior. Weight goes down, during a three month period, and glucose improves significantly.

This is just one more illustration that a person with type 2 diabetes has a better chance of controlling glucose by making sure that good weight levels are achieved and maintained.

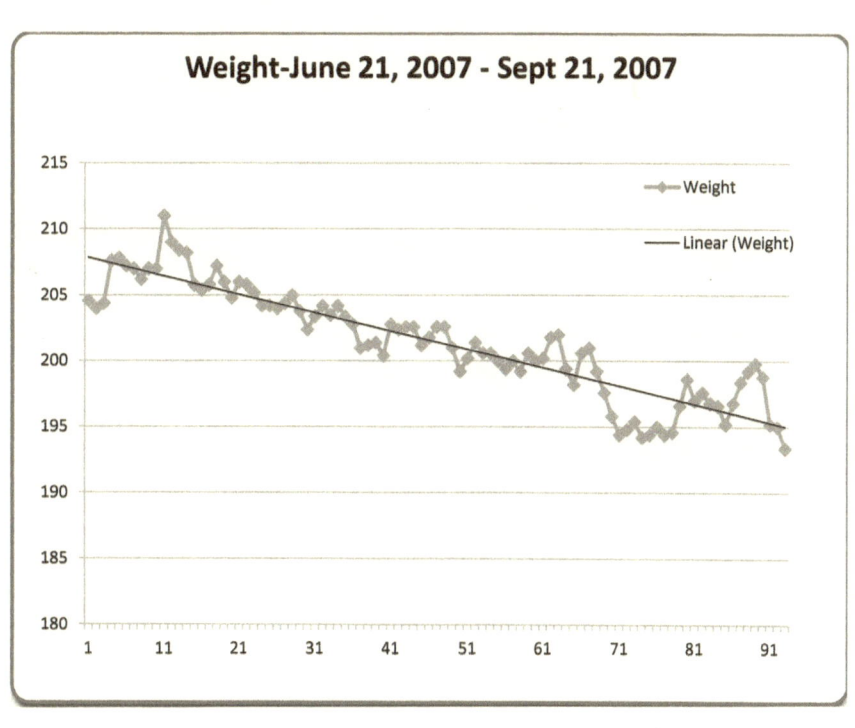

Weight-June 21, 2007 - Sept 21, 2007

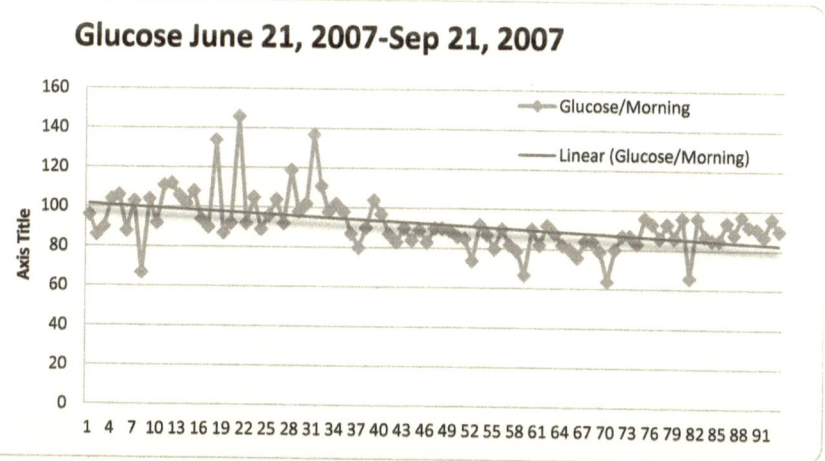

Glucose June 21, 2007-Sep 21, 2007

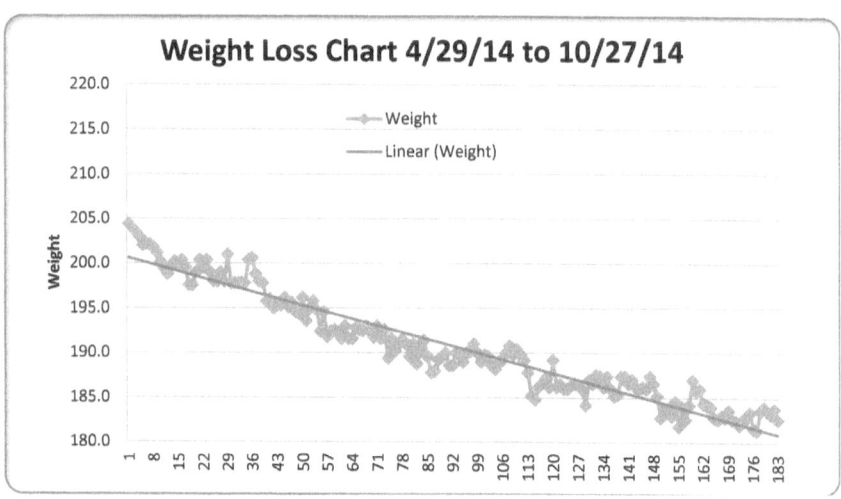

This is the most recent chart for weight management. This places me right where I want to be.

Diabetes Charts

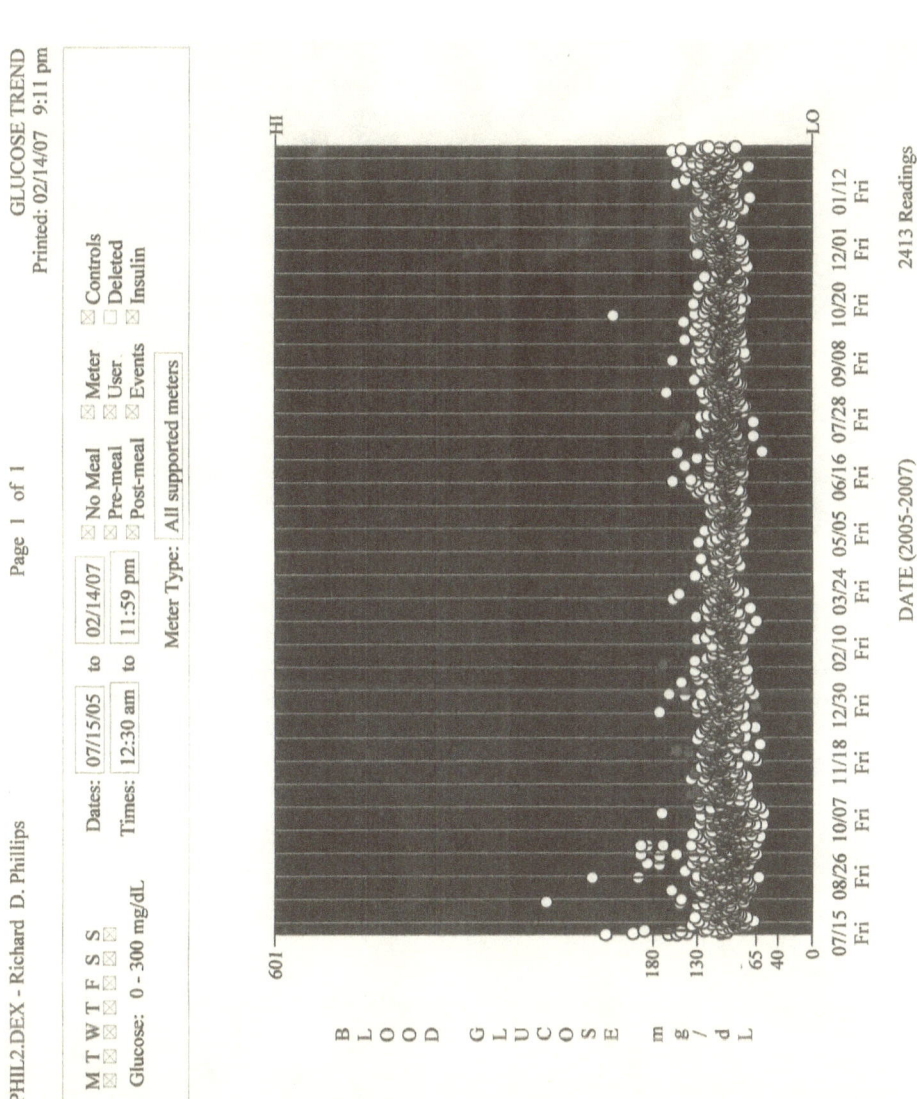

PHIL2.DEX - Richard D. Phillips   Page 1 of 1   GLUCOSE TREND
                                                                    Printed: 02/14/07 9:11 pm

M T W T F S S
☒ ☒ ☒ ☒ ☒ ☒ ☒
Glucose: 0 - 300 mg/dL

Dates: 07/15/05 to 02/14/07
Times: 12:30 am to 11:59 pm

☒ No Meal   ☒ Meter   ☒ Controls
☒ Pre-meal ☒ User.   ☐ Deleted
☒ Post-meal ☒ Events ☒ Insulin

Meter Type: All supported meters

BLOOD GLUCOSE mg/dL

601

HI

180
130
65
40
0

LO

07/15 08/26 10/07 11/18 12/30 02/10 03/24 05/05 06/16 07/28 09/08 10/20 12/01 01/12
Fri   Fri   Fri   Fri   Fri   Fri   Fri   Fri   Fri   Fri   Fri   Fri   Fri   Fri

DATE (2005-2007)   2413 Readings

133

Date	Time	Glucose	0	40	65		130	180		601	Comment
07/15/05 Fri	11:30 am	232 u							▪		First Metformin Half Tablet-500 mg
	11:30 am	E -									249.4 LBS
	4:00 pm	162 u						▪			Glipizide = 40 mg per day
	5:00 pm	152 u						▪			2nd Meformin Half Tablet 500 mg
	6:14 pm	E -									
07/16/05 Sat	11:30 am	202 u							▪		
	4:00 pm	141 u						▪			
	5:00 pm	104 u				▪					
	6:14 pm	E -									
07/17/05 Sun	12:01 pm	148 u						▪			
	4:00 pm	102 u				▪					
	5:00 pm	96 u				▪					
	6:14 pm	E -									
07/18/05 Mon	12:01 pm	189 u						▪			
	4:00 pm	122 u					▪				
	5:00 pm	110 u				▪					
	6:14 pm	E -									
07/19/05 Tue	12:01 pm	119 u					▪				
	4:00 pm	101 u				▪					
	5:00 pm	100 u				▪					
	6:14 pm	E -									
07/20/05 Wed	12:01 pm	94 u				▪					
	4:01 pm	89 u			▪						
	5:00 pm	86 u			▪						
	6:14 pm	E -									
07/21/05 Thu	12:01 pm	85 u			▪						
	4:00 pm	81 u			▪						
	5:00 pm	71 u			▪						
	6:14 pm	E -									
07/22/05 Fri	7:00 am	135 u					▪				
	7:00 am	E -									First Early Morning Reading

Date	Time	Glucose	0	40	65	130	180	601	Comment
07/22/05 Fri	7:00 am	E -							Dropped Daily Glipizide to 30 mg
	12:01 pm	74 u							
	5:00 pm	78 u							
	11:00 pm	88 u							
07/23/05 Sat	7:00 am	113 u							
	7:00 am	E -							Dropped Daily Glipizide to 20 mg
	12:01 pm	104 u							
	5:00 pm	87 u							
	11:00 pm	126 u							
07/24/05 Sun	7:00 am	123 u							
	11:45 am	67 u							
	5:00 pm	87 u							
	6:14 pm	E -							
	11:00 pm	98 u							
07/25/05 Mon	7:00 am	129 u							Split Glipizide to 10 mg am & pm
	7:00 am	E -							
	11:30 am	96 u							
	5:00 pm	78 u							2nd 10 mg Glipizide
	5:00 pm	E -							
	11:00 pm	89 u							
07/26/05 Tue	7:00 am	111 u							
	12:01 pm	90 u							
	5:00 pm	85 u							
	6:14 pm	E -							
	11:00 pm	79 u							
07/27/05 Wed	7:00 am	132 u							
	11:30 am	108 u							
	5:00 pm	107 u							
	6:14 pm	E -							
	11:00 pm	76 u							
07/28/05 Thu	7:00 am	108 u							244.4 LBS

Date	Time	Glucose	0	40	65	130	180	601	Comment
07/28/05 Thu	12:01 pm	90 u							
	5:00 pm	82 u							
	6:14 pm	E -							
	11:00 pm	109 u							
07/29/05 Fri	7:00 am	119 u							
	12:01 pm	108 u							
	5:00 pm	110 u							
	6:14 pm	E -							
	10:30 pm	82 u							
07/30/05 Sat	7:30 am	110 u							
	12:01 pm	85 u							
	5:00 pm	89 u							Took 5 mg Glipizide 5:00 pm
	5:00 pm	E -							Took 5 mg @ 11:00 pm
	10:30 pm	E -							
	11:00 pm	101 u							Glipizide change is working
07/31/05 Sun	7:00 am	92 u							
	7:00 am	E -							Un expected jump
	12:01 pm	118 u							
	12:01 pm	E -							
	5:00 pm	88 u							
	11:00 pm	108 u							
08/01/05 Mon	7:00 am	95 u							
	12:01 pm	96 u							
	5:00 pm	103 u							
	6:14 pm	E -							
	11:00 pm	88 u							
08/02/05 Tue	7:00 am	99 u							
	12:01 pm	96 u							
	5:00 pm	89 u							Accidentally took 10 mg Gl@ 5:00 pm
	6:14 pm	E -							
	11:00 pm	121 u							

Date	Time	Glucose	Comment
08/02/05 Tue	11:00 pm	E -	Took 5 mg GL @ 11:00 pm
08/03/05 Wed	7:00 am	114 u	
	12:01 pm	90 u	
	5:00 pm	90 u	
	6:14 pm	E -	
	11:00 pm	93 u	
08/04/05 Thu	7:00 am	107 u	
	12:01 pm	123 u	
	5:00 pm	94 u	
	6:14 pm	E -	
	11:00 pm	91 u	
08/05/05 Fri	7:00 am	113 u	
	12:01 pm	89 u	
	5:00 pm	94 u	
	5:00 pm	E -	Did not take 5 mg Glipizide 5:00 PM
	11:00 pm	130 u	Got burned- 11:00 PM too high
	11:03 pm	E -	
08/06/05 Sat	7:00 am	105 u	
	12:01 pm	102 u	
	5:00 pm	105 u	
	6:14 pm	E -	No Glipizide @ 5:00 PM
	11:00 pm	113 u	
	11:00 pm	E -	Cannot omit 5:00 PM Glipizide/5 mg
08/07/05 Sun	7:00 am	149 u	Cause unknown-way too high! New Dentures from yesterday?
	7:00 am	E -	
	7:00 am	E -	
	12:01 pm	122 u	
	5:00 pm	299 u	Partial Plate All Day today? Actual reading @ 306
	5:00 pm	E - S	
	11:00 pm	79 u	Back in conrol
	11:00 pm	E -	

Chart scale: 0 40 65 130 180 601

Date	Time	Glucose	0	40	65	130	180	601	Comment
08/08/05 Mon	7:00 am	106 u							
	12:01 pm	94 u							
	5:00 pm	102 u							
	11:00 pm	111 u							
	11:00 pm	E -							A Litle high @ bedtime
08/09/05 Tue	7:00 am	104 u							
	12:01 pm	101 u							
	5:00 pm	104 u							
	11:00 pm	148 u							Corn on the Cob & too much Fish
08/10/05 Wed	7:00 am	104 u							
	11:59 am	100 u							Back in control once again!
	12:03 pm	92 u							
	5:01 pm	88 u							
	9:30 pm	80 u							
08/11/05 Thu	7:15 am	99 u							
	12:15 am	94 u							
	5:00 pm	E -							2.5 mg Glipizide Only 5 Pm
	5:15 pm	93 u							
	8:00 pm	E -							2.5 mg Glipizide 8:00 P
	9:33 pm	101 u							
	11:00 pm	E -							5 mg Glipizide @ 11:00P
08/12/05 Fri	7:50 am	E -							
	7:51 am	117 u							
	12:15 pm	87 u							
	5:00 pm	107 u							
	11:05 pm	75 u							
08/13/05 Sat	5:34 am	91 u							
	6:15 am	E - D							Ate Breakfast @ 6:15 am
	9:00 am	78 u							
	9:15 am	E -							Took 2 Glucose tablets-running low
	12:15 pm	125 u							

Date	Time	Glucose	0	40	65	130	180	601	Comment
08/13/05 Sat	3:09 pm	E - D							Ate Small Lunch-tomatoes-Zucchini
	5:10 pm	94 u							
	9:45 pm	113 u							
08/14/05 Sun	8:15 am	E - S							
	12:10 pm	126 u							500 mg met & 10 mg Glip / Unusual-should be dropping
	5:45 pm	80 u							
	5:45 pm	E -							looking Good took 5 mg + 500 mg / Looking good-Raisins/apricot / Raisins-night before-
	8:46 pm	88 u							
08/15/05 Mon	6:32 am	125 u							
	11:00 am	126 u							
	12:10 pm	111 u							
	5:30 pm	86 u							
	5:30 pm	E - S							2.5 mG Glipizide @ 5:30 PM / Looking Good-2.5 mg Glipizide 8:30
	8:30 pm	81 u							
	9:06 pm	78 u							
	11:30 pm	E - S							2.5 Glipizide @11:30 PM
	11:35 pm	99 u							
08/16/05 Tue	7:58 am	101 u							Excellent Start / Eggs for breakfast
	12:02 pm	81 u							
	3:30 pm	86 u							
	5:30 pm	87 u							2.5 mg Glipizide @ Dinner / Glucose on target all day
	6:56 pm	E -							
	8:30 pm	96 u							
	9:30 pm	99 u							Ate Pudding took 2.5 mg Glipizide / Took last 5 mg Glipizide-Unusual hi / Held up Glipizide too long
	11:58 pm	159 u							A little High
	11:58 pm	E -							took too much Glip at 20 mg Yesterd
08/17/05 Wed	1:45 am	117 u							Took 1 Glucose Tablet @ 4:00 am
	4:00 am	70 u							Levels dropping-Normal Pattern
	4:00 am	E -							
	11:39 am	90 u							

Date	Time	Glucose	0	40	65	130	180	601	Comment
08/17/05 Wed	3:50 pm	113 u							5 mg Glip+Met & ate late supper
	6:30 pm	87 u							2.5 mg Glipizide-Scrambled eggs
	10:30 pm	85 u							Eggs & Nuts @ 10:30 + 2.5 mg glip
08/18/05 Thu	12:35 am	82 u							
	4:25 am	85 u							
	6:00 am	110 u							
	9:55 am	70 u							Late Breakfast
	12:30 pm	114 u							
	2:30 pm	96 u							
	5:25 pm	99 u							Diet Ice cream 2.5 mg Glip
	9:30 pm	101 u							On Target @ 88
	10:30 pm	88 u							Will not stop work until 2 :00 AM
08/19/05 Fri	1:06 am	73 u							
	1:56 am	78 u							
	6:24 am	85 u							
	11:30 am	119 u							Breakfast fried food & hash browns
	11:30 am	E -							
	12:30 pm	114 u							
	4:30 pm	96 u							Forgot Medicine-took after meal
	6:00 pm	91 u							Hamburger Patty-No bread
	6:00 pm	E -							Yellow Squash/Dinner
	9:30 pm	122 u							
	10:30 pm	81 u							Too High 10 mg Glip 8:45a
08/20/05 Sat	8:45 am	122 u							Still a little high @ Lunch Time
	12:42 pm	109 u							OOPS!
	3:30 pm	132 u							2.5 Glipizide 5:25p+dinner
	5:25 pm	96 u							2.5 mg Glipizide 8:15 p
	8:15 pm	85 u							Small diet ice cream 8:15p.........
	8:15 pm	E -							2.5 mg Glip + 3/4 Glass of milk
	11:05 pm	108 u							Looks Good
08/21/05 Sun	1:49 am	100 u							

Date	Time	Glucose	0	40	65	130	180	601	Comment
08/21/05 Sun	2:40 am	109 u							
	3:35 am	104 u							Early meds help!
	8:25 am	95 u							Great!
	12:15 pm	83 u							Late Lunch
	1:30 pm	103 u							Luncheon-1 hot dog +tomatoes-chili
	6:00 pm	116 u							
	6:00 pm	E -							2.5 Glip @ 6:00 P
	9:30 pm	73 u							Grapenuts 2.5 mg Glip @ 9:30 PM
	11:10 pm	E -							2.5 MG Glip @ 11:10p
08/22/05 Mon	8:00 am	130 u							Too High-Yesterday's diet violated
	9:55 am	115 u							
	1:10 pm	132 u							
	4:00 pm	78 u							
	5:40 pm	78 u							
	9:00 pm	85 u							
08/23/05 Tue	9:00 am	126 u							
	1:00 pm	81 u							
	4:50 pm	130 u							
	7:45 pm	75 u							
08/24/05 Wed	12:30 am	116 u							Drove Through SB/Cycle
	7:20 am	129 u							Ate Banana & Peanut Butter
	12:15 pm	111 u							Only took total 15 mg/day yesterday
	6:00 pm	96 u							
	9:05 pm	95 u							
	10:00 pm	96 u							Zucchini+small pc loaf
08/25/05 Thu	1:15 am	116 u							
	7:45 am	106 u							
	12:15 pm	100 u							
	5:30 pm	79 u							Looking Good!
	9:35 pm	87 u							
08/26/05 Fri	2:00 am	196 u							Forgot Last Night's medicine-Glipiz

Date	Time	Glucose	0	40	65	130	180	601	Comment
08/26/05 Fri	4:20 am	248 u							Ate Berries @ 10:pm Snack-no med
	5:50 am	125 u							Much Better-back on track
	9:00 am	62 u							A Little Low-but OK
	1:30 pm	130 u							Overcompensated with raisins
	2:30 pm	120 u							
	5:30 pm	87 u							
	9:30 pm	104 u							
08/27/05 Sat	7:15 am	99 u							Fresh Tomato-Zucchini
	12:05 pm	104 u							Baked Fish
	4:30 pm	96 u							Diet Jello
	8:30 pm	92 u							
	10:45 pm	92 u							
08/28/05 Sun	8:30 am	100 u							
	12:15 pm	99 u							
	5:30 pm	92 u							
	9:00 pm	102 u							
	11:10 pm	99 u							
08/29/05 Mon	5:00 am	87 u							Bob Evans Cajun Catfish @5:30
	6:30 am	113 u							1.5 Garlic Bread @ Bob Evans 5:30
	8:15 am	100 u							
	12:16 pm	113 u							
	5:00 pm	98 u							
	8:30 pm	117 u							
	9:30 pm	109 u							
08/30/05 Tue	8:00 am	120 u							Late Lunch-tomatoes
	9:20 am	110 u							Early Dinner-Beans/Nuts
	2:30 pm	92 u							Unexpected High-Pos Stress
	4:45 pm	88 u							
	8:15 pm	144 u							
	9:00 pm	118 u							
	9:45 pm	104 u							Ate Small Snack-eggs 9:45p

Date	Time	Glucose	0	40	65	130	180	601	Comment
08/30/05 Tue	11:05 pm	83 u							Back on Target
08/31/05 Wed	5:45 am	99 u							500 Met & 10 Glip
	6:30 am	97 u							Took Glucose Tablet
	10:00 am	80 u							No Breakfast-Took Glucose Tablet
	12:15 pm	87 u							
	4:40 pm	115 u							500 Met & 2.5 Glip
	5:25 pm	99 u							Beans & Spinach
	8:30 pm	105 u							Diet Ice Cream + 2.5 Glip
09/01/05 Thu	4:10 am	85 u							Looking Great!
	5:15 am	100 u							500 Met 10 Glip
	9:50 am	92 u							
	10:50 am	90 u							
	6:00 pm	92 u							
	6:00 pm	E-							At Indy Hospital/Dean
	9:00 pm	88 u							500 Met 2.5 Glip/Roasted Chicken
	10:00 pm	113 u							2.5 Glip-Chicken Snack
09/02/05 Fri	7:30 am	E - S							7:30 2.5 Glip-Forgot last night
	8:00 am	94 u							500 Met + 10 Glip
	9:00 am	79 u							Late Breakfast
	12:15 pm	74 u							Tending Neighbor's Dogs
	5:01 pm	83 u							Roasted Chicken-Salad-Tomato + meds
	6:30 pm	75 u							Banana & Raisins/Peanut Butter
	8:30 pm	118 u							2.5 Glip
	11:20 pm	122 u							2.5 Glip
09/03/05 Sat	3:00 am	82 u							
	4:00 am	73 u							500 Met 10 Glip
	8:15 am	93 u							Moving office-tending dogs
	12:10 pm	82 u							Roast Chicken For Lunch
	12:10 pm	E-							moving office all day
	3:45 pm	84 u							2.5 glip 500 met hamgurger/spinach
	5:15 pm	86 u							

Date	Time	Glucose	0	40	65	130	180	601	Comment
09/03/05 Sat	6:25 pm	76 u							1 glucose tablet
	8:20 pm	87 u							
	10:45 pm	106 u							2.5 Glip
	10:47 pm	E -							Only took 15 mg glip today
09/04/05 Sun	6:30 am	106 u							Only took 15 glip yesterday
	6:30 am	E -							10 glip 500 met @ 6:30 am
	9:05 am	130 u							Church Performance-Guitar/Vocal
	10:30 am	122 u							Stress Probable
	12:45 pm	173 u							Stress-Deacon's-Meeting-Red Cross
	12:45 pm	E -							5 mg Glip
	6:30 pm	73 u							Back on Track
	9:30 pm	85 u							
	11:00 pm	116 u							Drank a Glass of milk
09/05/05 Mon	7:30 am	123 u							A Little high for the start
	7:30 am	E -							500 Met 10 Glip-usual Dosage
	9:00 am	116 u							Still Too high
	12:15 pm	106 u							Still a little high
	5:30 pm	98 u							500 Met+ 2.5 Glip
	8:30 pm	186 u							Chicago Pizza-Major error!
	9:30 pm	136 u							Improving- 5 mg Glip
	11:15 pm	123 u							2.5 Glip-improving
09/06/05 Tue	7:45 am	97 u							On Target
	11:40 am	84 u							
	5:10 pm	84 u							
	8:05 pm	95 u							Outstanding 500 Met 2.5 Glip
	11:10 pm	115 u							
09/07/05 Wed	12:30 am	108 u							2.5 glip
	1:30 am	109 u							
	7:45 am	95 u							
	11:45 am	77 u							
	4:30 pm	98 u							

Date	Time	Glucose	0	40	65	130	180	601	Comment
09/07/05 Wed	5:15 pm	88 u							2.5 Glip-Stress/Council Meeting
	9:00 pm	130 u							Back On Track
	11:30 pm	86 u							
09/08/05 Thu	12:30 am	84 u							
	1:30 am	78 u							
	7:30 am	101 u							500 mg Met 10 mg Glip eggs
	10:20 am	77 u							Great- May Reduce morning meds
	11:30 am	86 u							
	3:30 pm	90 u							
	5:00 pm	82 u							
	5:30 pm	87 u							500 met 2.5 glip
	8:30 pm	115 u							Hard Biking 2.5 Glip
	11:00 pm	87 u							Back On Track
09/09/05 Fri	12:30 am	76 u							
	1:10 am	86 u							500 met 10 Glip -- Eggs
	8:15 am	95 u							Drove Cycle to VA in Marion
	11:30 am	80 u							Tomatoes
	12:45 pm	69 u							Eating Piece Stawberry Diet Pie
	3:15 pm	80 u							500 Met 2.5 Glip- see 3:15 note
	5:15 pm	127 u							Looking Good
	7:30 pm	93 u							Pudding & 2.5 Glip
	10:15 pm	97 u							2.5 Glip
	11:30 pm	123 u							
09/10/05 Sat	5:15 pm	106 u							Good Start 500 Met 10 Glip
	6:10 am	85 u							Family Reunion-music-announcing
	7:25 am	85 u							500 met 2.5 glip
	12:15 pm	103 u							Ate beans & 2 hamburger patties-fat
	4:55 pm	88 u							very unusual-ate banana
	6:00 pm	p 85 u							Ate a piece of SF Stawberry pie
	7:30 pm	76 u P							
	8:30 pm	E -							

Date	Time	Glucose	0	40	65	130	180	601	Comment
09/10/05 Sat	9:35 pm	134 u							2.5 glip-SF Straweberry Pie&Banana
	11:30 pm	173 u							2.5 Glip-surprised so hi-Pie/Burger
09/11/05 Sun	4:00 am	71 u							Back on track-a little low
	8:00 am	87 u							500 Met 10 Glip
	12:00 pm	p 86 u							On Target
	4:00 pm	85 u							
	5:00 pm	E - T							Heavy EQ lifting-Long Hauling
	7:00 pm	E - T							Heavy EQ Lifting-Long hauling
	7:30 pm	p 155 u							500 Met 2.5 Glip-Duke's CC Show
	9:30 pm	193 u P							2.5 Glip Meds Late-ate late @ 7:30
	11:30 pm	154 u							2.5 Glip-Public Appearance
09/12/05 Mon	2:10 am	67 u							OK-a little low-Glucose Tablet
	7:30 am	92 u							500 met 10 glip
	9:20 am	65 u P							1 Glucose Tablet
	12:15 pm	p 77 u							
	4:00 pm	76 u							1 Glucose Tablet
	5:20 pm	87 u							500 Met 2.5 Glip
	8:45 pm	p 80 u							Super Day 2.5 Glip
	11:00 pm	108 u P							
09/13/05 Tue	7:00 am	108 u P							500 Met & Only 7.5 Glip
	9:50 am	80 u P							Excellent Result
	11:15 am	72 u							
	2:40 pm	94 u P							
	5:20 pm	p 90 u							500 met 2.5 glip
	6:50 pm	86 u P							chicken/spinach/peas @5:20pm
	8:30 pm	82 u							Small Amount of Berries snack
	10:45 pm	92 u							Only took 10 mg Glip today!
09/14/05 Wed	6:30 am	p 97 u							500 Met 7.5 Glip @6:45 am
	7:00 am	E -							Breakfast-2 eggs
	9:00 am	69 u P							
	11:15 am	77 u							Banana

Date	Time	Glucose	0	40	65	130	180	601	Comment
09/14/05 Wed	3:30 pm	114 u							500 Met 2.5 Glip
	5:20 pm	p 97 u							
	9:30 pm	89 u							
	10:45 pm	93 u							2.5 Glip
09/15/05 Thu	8:00 am	109 u							500 Met 7.5 Glip
	11:55 am	87 u							On Track
	4:45 pm	110 u							Bill's Funeral 2.5 Glip 500 Metfor
	5:45 pm	109 u							Lion Hog Roast Activity
	8:35 pm	110 u							2.5 Glip-Late dinner
09/16/05 Fri	7:50 am	102 u							7.5 Glip & 500 Met
	11:35 am	86 u							
	12:40 pm	86 u							2.5 Glip 500 Met
	5:15 pm	85 u							May have forgot Glip & Met/Dinner
	5:15 pm	100 u							2.5 Glip-Preparing For Art Show
	8:30 pm	126 u							
	10:10 pm	80 u							
	11:10 pm	75 u							
09/17/05 Sat	3:50 am	80 u							7.5 Glip 500 Met
	7:10 am	103 u							
	12:05 pm	84 u							2.5 Glip 500 Met
	4:30 pm	78 u							Great!
	8:30 pm	82 u							2.5 Glip 500 Met
	9:35 pm	81 u							Diet Ice Cream/Banana Snack
09/18/05 Sun	7:20 am	85 u							2.5 Glip 500 Met
	12:05 pm	113 u							NJ @ MBC
	1:30 pm	186 u							NJ @ Paradise Park
	2:45 pm	193 u							Migraine- Lasted about 1 hour
	2:45 pm	E - IST							2.5 Glip
	3:30 pm	E - 168 u							
	5:15 pm	102 u							2.5 Glip 500 Met

147

Date	Time	Glucose	0	40	65	130	180	601	Comment
09/18/05 Sun	7:30 pm	69 u							Banana/Nuts/Peanut Butter
09/19/05 Mon	11:30 pm	137 u							2.5 Glip
	8:15 am	96 u							7.5 Glip 500 Met
	12:05 pm	102 u							
	4:10 pm	89 u							2.5 Glip 500 Met
	7:15 pm	101 u							
	8:30 pm	86 u							
	9:30 pm	86 u							
	10:25 pm	88 u							
09/20/05 Tue	8:15 am	122 u							500 Met 7.5 Glip-Accucheck
	3:30 pm	86 u							
	4:30 pm	83 u							
	5:30 pm	E -							2.5 Glip 500 Met
	6:20 pm	E -							2.5 Glip Peanut Butter/Raisins
	8:10 pm	64 u							
	8:30 pm	75 u							
	11:15 pm	124 u							2.5 Glip
09/21/05 Wed	6:00 am	96 u							Last Strip/Accucheck
	6:32 am	91 u							New Strips 500 Met 5mg Glip
	11:30 am	120 u							2.5 Glip
	3:30 pm	101 u							
	5:00 pm	96 u							500 Met 2.5 Glip
	9:15 pm	118 u							
	10:35 pm	117 u							2.5 Glip
09/22/05 Thu	6:30 am	96 u							500 Met 7.5 Glip
	12:05 pm	110 u							
	5:15 pm	101 u							2.5 Glip 500 Met
	9:00 pm	100 u							
	11:00 pm	100 u							2.5 glip
09/23/05 Fri	7:45 am	91 u							500 Met 7.5 Glip
	11:45 am	87 u							

Date	Time	Glucose	0	40	65	130	180	601	Comment
09/23/05 Fri	4:30 pm	105 u							500 Met 2.5 Glip
	7:05 pm	76 u							Chicken-Spinach
	10:00 pm	100 u							2.5 glip
09/24/05 Sat	3:45 am	126 u							
	7:50 am	97 u							7.5 Glip & 500 Met
	12:00 pm	87 u							
	4:20 pm	92 u							Reli-On Meter-Ultima
	5:05 pm	81 u							2.5 Glip 500 Met
	8:55 pm	81 u							Third reading-Ultima
	10:10 pm	p 86 u P							
09/25/05 Sun	3:20 am	98 u							Ultima May Read Low
	4:15 am	99 u							Meas Ultima with Elite-Verified
	5:40 am	107 u							2.5 Glip-Verified
	7:10 am	p 93 u							95/Elite 7.5 Glip 500 Met
	9:00 am	60 u							1 Glucose Tablet-Too Low-Verified
	10:20 am	75 u							Verified
	11:15 am	p 77 u							
	1:00 pm	E -							Ate About 1:00 pm
	3:30 pm	97 u P							
	5:00 pm	93 u							2.5 Glip 500 Met
	7:30 pm	131 u							BD-Diet Pie/Diet Ice Cream @ 6:00
	7:30 pm	E -							2.5 Glip
	8:00 pm	106 u							
	9:00 pm	100 u							
	10:20 pm	70 u							Snack
09/26/05 Mon	5:30 am	105 u							
	8:00 am	99 u							Ham & Beans
	11:50 am	98 u							2.5 Glip 500 Met
	5:00 pm	109 u							2.5 Glip
	8:30 pm	135 u							7.5 Glip 500 Met
09/27/05 Tue	7:10 am	105 u							

Date	Time	Glucose	0	40	65	130	180	601	Comment
09/27/05 Tue	8:10 am	116 u							
	11:10 am	92 u							
	4:30 pm	97 u							2.5 Glip 500 Met
	5:15 pm	E - D							Dinner @ 5:15 pm
	9:05 pm	95 u							
09/28/05 Wed	6:30 am	p 107 u							7.5 Glip 500 Met
	9:45 am	87 u P							Elite
	11:20 am	97 u							
	3:10 pm	96 u							Great
	5:15 pm	101 u							
	9:15 pm	94 u							
09/29/05 Thu	8:00 am	p 113 u							Late Breakfast 7.5 Glip 500 Met
	8:35 am	E -							
	11:15 am	100 u P							
	1:00 pm	96 u							Late Lunch
	5:45 pm	102 u							2.5 Glip 500 Met
	7:45 pm	70 u							
	8:30 pm	80 u							
	9:20 pm	83 u							
09/30/05 Fri	1:10 am	99 u							Pudding
	6:30 am	p 83 u							Looking Good
	9:50 am	76 u P							7.5 Glip 500 Met
	11:20 am	96 u							Exercise-bike-shop remodel
	12:00 pm	97 u							
	4:45 pm	101 u							
	6:45 pm	81 u P							
	8:05 pm	84 u							
10/01/05 Sat	6:45 am	83 u							
	7:45 am	p E -							
	8:30 am	p 100 u							7.5 Glip 500 Met
	9:45 am	65 u P							

Date	Time	Glucose	0	40	65	130	180	601	Comment
10/01/05 Sat	11:00 am	E -							
	11:55 am	p 77 u							
	4:05 pm	87 u							Glucose Tablet
	7:35 pm	78 u P							
	7:46 pm	E -							
	8:40 pm	80 u							500 met 2.5 glip Banana/peanut butter/peanuts
10/02/05 Sun	7:35 am	105 u							500 Met 7.5 Glip
	12:30 pm	83 u							
	5:50 pm	85 u							500 Met 2.5 Glip
	7:00 pm	74 u P							222 Lbs
	9:00 pm	83 u							
	11:10 pm	90 u							
10/03/05 Mon	7:50 am	99 u							500 Met 7.5 glip Glucose Tablet
	10:10 am	57 u P							Will Reduce met or Glip tomorrow Glucose tablet
	10:20 am	E -							Glucose Tablet
	11:50 am	p 66 u							
	1:05 pm	83 u P							
	5:29 pm	79 u							500 Met 2.5 Glip
	6:15 pm	p 85 u							
	9:00 pm	110 u							
	10:00 pm	93 u							
10/04/05 Tue	2:00 am	112 u							
	4:30 pm	115 u							5.0 glip 500 met Exercise–biking
	6:00 am	E -							
	7:10 am	p 127 u							
	11:00 am	97 u							
	12:00 pm	p 94 u							
	2:55 pm	111 uc P							Reduced Glipizide This AM
	3:35 pm	103 u							
	9:00 pm	100 u							
	11:05 pm	95 u							

Date	Time	Glucose	0	40	65	130	180	601	Comment
10/05/05 Wed	7:50 am	p 105 u							5.0 Glip 500 Met
	10:45 am	73 u P							
	12:15 pm	77 u							
	5:40 pm	p 98 u							2.5 Glip 500 met
	7:55 pm	76 u P							Great!
	8:25 pm	87 u							Switched to Accucheck Meter
10/06/05 Thu	6:30 am	p 88 u							
	7:05 am	p E -							5 Glip. 500 Met 1/2 Atenolol
	11:30 am	87 u							
	12:05 pm	97 u							
	3:50 pm	88 u							
	5:05 pm	p 83 u							500 Met 2.5 Glip
	7:40 pm	84 u							
	11:15 pm	98 u							
10/07/05 Fri	7:30 am	p 96 u							5 Glip & 500 Met & 1/2 Atenolol
	10:30 am	84 u P							Ate About 8:00 AM
	12:20 pm	p 87 u							
	4:40 pm	p 91 u							
	8:20 pm	86 u							2.5 glip 500 met
	10:10 pm	108 u							
10/08/05 Sat	4:35 pm	107 u							
	6:00 am	p 124 u							5 Glip 500 Met 1/2 Atenolol
	7:30 am	p 88 u							
	10:20 am	99 u P							
	11:45 am	p 102 u							
	3:25 pm	113 u							
	4:35 pm	102 u							
	5:05 pm	p 104 u							2.5 Glip 500 Met
	8:30 pm	108 u P							Food tasting Part-Dentures
	9:00 pm	108 u							
10/09/05 Sun	7:30 am	p 117 u							5 Glip 500 Met

152

Date	Time	Glucose	0	40	65	130	180	601	Comment
10/09/05 Sun	12:35 pm	p 90 u							
	8:45 pm	p 100 u							2.5 Glip 500 Met Late meal
	10:40 pm	126 u P							
10/10/05 Mon	7:20 am	95 u							5 glip 500 Met 1/2 Atenolol
	10:10 am	p 71 u							Forgot to eat breakfast- ate 10:10
	12:05 pm	p 82 u							
	3:45 pm	90 u							
	5:25 pm	p 101 u							500 met 2.5 glip
	8:40 pm	84 u							
10/11/05 Tue	7:45 am	p 109 u							5 glip 500 met 1/2 Atenolol
	9:25 am	66 u P							Ate about 8:30 AM
	12:05 pm	p 82 u							
	5:15 pm	p 86 u							2.5 Glip 500 Met
	8:10 pm	71 u P							Exercise Stepped up
	11:10 pm	170 u							Diet Pudding With banana & nuts 9pm
	11:10 pm	E -							Extra 2.5 glip to counter goof!
10/12/05 Wed	12:35 am	114 u							
	8:10 am	p 79 u							5 glip 500 met
	10:09 am	56 u P							Glucose Tablet
	12:05 pm	p 91 u							
	3:15 pm	83 u P							
	5:05 pm	p 86 u							2.5 glip 500 met
	7:25 pm	70 u P							
	10:20 pm	99 u							
10/13/05 Thu	4:05 am	83 u							Snacked @ 8 banana & Nuts
	6:30 am	p 94 u							
	9:45 am	69 u							
	12:00 pm	p 84 u							2.5 glip 500 Met
	2:00 pm	107 u							
	3:45 pm	87 u							
	5:00 pm	82 u							

Date	Time	Glucose	0	40	65	130	180	601	Comment
10/13/05 Thu	8:00 pm	107 u P							Snack-Only took 2.5 Glip for the da
	9:00 pm	101 u							
	11:05 pm	106 u							
10/14/05 Fri	12:35 am	114 uc							2.5 Glip Yesterday!!!!
	1:40 am	100 u							
	7:55 am	p 97 u							2.5 Glip 500 Met
	12:15 pm	p 95 u							
	4:30 pm	p 96 u							500 Met 0 Glip
	8:05 pm	100 u P							
10/15/05 Sat	4:30 am	96 u							2.5 glip 500 met
	7:40 am	p 108 u							Late Breakfast
	9:30 am	p E -							
	11:10 am	67 u P							
	12:40 pm	87 u							
	4:50 pm	p 95 u							500 met
	8:30 pm	104 u P							
	10:30 pm	112 u P							
10/16/05 Sun	7:50 am	p 103 u							
	12:15 pm	p 115 u							
	5:30 pm	p 92 u							
	8:15 pm	100 u							
	10:40 pm	104 u							
10/17/05 Mon	7:30 am	p 86 u							500 Met 2.5 Glip
	9:55 am	60 u P							
	12:00 pm	99 u							
	2:50 pm	88 u							
	5:00 pm	p 86 u							500 met
	8:05 pm	105 u P							
	11:55 pm	128 u							
10/18/05 Tue	8:10 am	p 90 u							500 Met 2.5 Glip
	9:35 am	66 u P							

154

Date	Time	Glucose	0	40	65	130	180	601	Comment
10/18/05 Tue	12:10 pm	p 87 u			▪				
	4:05 pm	86 u			▪				
	5:45 pm	p 89 u			▪				500 Met
	9:00 pm	93 u			▪				Diet Jello/Nuts
10/19/05 Wed	7:20 am	p 79 u			▪				2.5 Glip 500 Met
	9:05 am	77 u P			▪				
	10:00 am	70 u P		▪					Took Glucose Tab-Ballparked reading
	12:30 pm	p 80 u			▪				
	3:25 pm	94 u P			▪				
	5:15 pm	p 84 u			▪				500 met
	9:15 pm	85 u			▪				
10/20/05 Thu	7:30 am	p 84 uc			▪				500 Met Only-No Glip
	10:45 am	99 u P			▪				
	12:10 pm	p 101 u				▪			
	3:30 pm	p 91 u			▪				500 Met
	8:10 pm	p 88 u			▪				
	10:45 pm	108 u P				▪			Snacked-Boiled Chick/nuts/pie diet
	10:45 pm	E -							No Glipizide For The day!
10/21/05 Fri	7:30 am	p 85 u			▪				500 Met
	11:10 am	107 u				▪			
	3:10 pm	99 u P			▪				
	5:10 pm	p 82 u			▪				500 Met
	8:20 pm	102 u				▪			
	11:05 pm	128 u				▪			
10/22/05 Sat	7:30 am	p 105 u				▪			500 Met
	12:05 pm	p 109 u				▪			Ultima
	4:00 pm	107 u				▪			Elite
	4:45 pm	p 95 u			▪				Elite
	7:40 pm	113 u P				▪			Elite
10/23/05 Sun	7:30 am	p 103 u				▪			500 Met - Elite
	12:00 pm	p 125 u				▪			

Date	Time	Glucose	Comment
10/23/05 Sun	6:20 pm	p 104 u	500 Met
	8:05 pm	129 u P	
	11:05 pm	110 u	
10/24/05 Mon	2:40 am	113 u	
	8:15 am	p 105 u	500 Met
	11:55 am	p 130 u	
	4:10 pm	110 u	
	5:30 pm	p 106 u	500 Met / Small Snack-Peanut Butter/Banana
	9:00 pm	E -	
	9:55 pm	p 105 u P	500 Met
10/25/05 Tue	7:30 am	p 100 u	2.5 Glip
	12:24 pm	p 137 uc	
	5:10 pm	p 76 u	
	9:30 pm	121 u	
	11:25 pm	128 u P	
10/26/05 Wed	5:25 pm	p 113 u	Late Break 500 Met
	8:10 am	p E -	2.5 Glip
	10:00 am	137 uc P	
	12:00 pm	p 83 u	
	3:00 pm	88 u P	
	5:50 pm	p 83 u	500 Met
	9:15 pm	95 u	
10/27/05 Thu	5:15 pm	106 u	
	8:00 am	p 110 u	500 Met 2.5 Glip
	12:15 pm	92 u	
	4:30 pm	95 u	
	9:30 pm	p 110 u	
10/28/05 Fri	8:00 am	p 99 u	Board Meeting / 500 Met 2.5 Glip
	12:10 pm	98 u	
	3:40 pm	117 u	
	6:15 pm	p 103 u	500 Met

Chart axis markers: 0 40 65 130 180 601

156

Date	Time	Glucose	0	40	65	130	180	601	Comment
10/28/05 Fri	9:45 pm	104 u							
10/29/05 Sat	1:30 am	129 u							Unusually High-No Explanation
	2:00 am	130 uc							2.5 Glip to Lower
	3:30 am	120 u							
	8:10 am	p 75 u							
	12:00 pm	107 u							
	4:15 pm	104 u							Clara Wouster's funeral
	6:10 pm	p 97 u							
	11:59 pm	115 uc							A Guess- Actual time 12:50 AM
10/30/05 Sun	12:50 am	115 u							
	8:00 am	p 114 u							500 Met 2.5 Glip
	12:00 pm	p 119 u							PA
									500 Met
	5:30 pm	p 108 u							500 met 2.5 glip
10/31/05 Mon	6:10 am	111 u							
	8:50 am	p 81 u							
	11:10 am	96 u							
	1:10 pm	p 95 u							Plugged
	5:10 pm	p 88 u							500 met
	8:50 pm	117 u P							
	10:45 pm	99 u							
11/01/05 Tue	8:00 am	p 104 u							500 Met 2.5 Glip
	10:30 am	79 u P							
	11:40 am	94 u P							
	2:45 pm	103 u P							
	5:00 pm	p 94 u							500 Met
	8:50 pm	112 u							
	11:00 pm	103 u							
11/02/05 Wed	7:30 am	p 102 u							500 Met 2.5 Glip
	9:10 am	74 u P							
	12:30 pm	p 105 u							
	5:00 pm	81 u							500 Met

Date	Time	Glucose	0	40	65	130	180	601	Comment
11/02/05 Wed	6:15 pm	p 92 u							500 met 2.5 glip
11/03/05 Thu	7:30 am	p 99 u							
	12:15 pm	p 106 u							500 met
	5:05 pm	p 91 u							
	9:10 pm	103 u P							
11/04/05 Fri	7:30 am	p 104 u							500 met 2.5 glip
	12:10 pm	p 96 u							
	3:05 pm	100 u P							500 met
	4:35 pm	E -							500 Met
	5:55 pm	p E - S							
11/05/05 Sat	4:30 am	124 u							500 met 2.5 glip
	7:00 am	107 u							
	9:30 am	p 92 u							
	9:30 am	100 u							
	2:55 pm	p 88 u							500 Met
	5:55 pm	p E - S							500 met
	6:30 pm	E -							
11/06/05 Sun	8:40 pm	p 96 u							500 met 2.5 glip
	7:10 am	p 110 u							Ate Breakfast-eggs
	8:10 am	p E -							
	9:10 am	79 u P							Try 1.25 AM/PM Glip 11 7 05
	9:10 am	E - S							
	12:40 pm	p 97 u							500 Met
	5:55 pm	p E - S							Public Appearance-Gilead
	9:25 pm	119 u							
	11:55 pm	137 u P							500 Met 1.25 Glip
11/07/05 Mon	8:30 am	117 u							
	12:15 pm	p 96 u							500 met
	5:20 pm	p 122 u							
	9:30 pm	91 u							
	11:55 pm	100 u P							

158

Date	Time	Glucose	0	40	65	130	180	601	Comment
11/08/05 Tue	8:00 am	p 99 uc							500 Met 1.25 Glip
	11:00 am	76 u							
	12:10 pm	p 96 u							
	5:55 pm	p 102 u							500 Met
	8:25 pm	98 u							
	11:05 pm	105 u P							
11/09/05 Wed	7:15 am	102 uc							1.25 Glip 500 Met
	8:25 am	p 82 u							
	1:15 pm	p 100 u							
	6:00 pm	p 102 u							500 Met
	9:00 pm	98 u P							
	11:55 pm	110 u P							
11/10/05 Thu	6:36 am	105 u P							500 Met 1.25 Glip - Weighed 210.6
	8:00 am	p 94 u							
	10:10 am	97 u P							
	12:10 pm	p 82 u							
	2:30 pm	96 u P							
	5:20 pm	p 96 u							Forgot Metformin
	6:30 pm	E - S P							500 Metformin
	9:30 pm	106 u P							
11/11/05 Fri	6:10 am	118 u							Took 500 Met 1.25 Glip
	6:25 am	E - S							
	9:00 am	p 87 u							
	12:00 pm	p 133 uc							1.25 glip
	4:00 pm	87 u							
	5:25 pm	p 89 u							500 Met
	10:44 pm	117 u P							Mary's Party
11/12/05 Sat	8:00 am	p 99 u							500 Met 1.25 Glip
	12:30 pm	p 108 u							
	5:50 pm	p 113 u							
	9:25 pm	p 112 u							Tokk med very Late

Date	Time	Glucose	0	40	65	130	180	601	Comment
11/12/05 Sat	11:55 pm	116 u							500 Met 1.25 Glip
11/13/05 Sun	8:00 am	p 105 u							Forgot to take reading
	12:00 pm	p E -							500 Met
	4:00 pm	p 105 u							
	9:15 pm	p 110 u							
11/14/05 Mon	3:15 am	115 u							500 met 1.25 glip
	8:00 am	p 106 u							Forgot to eat breakfast
	9:20 am	p 106 u							
	12:00 pm	p 117 u							
	6:55 pm	p 102 u							500 met
	9:15 pm	126 u P							
11/15/05 Tue	8:00 am	114 u							500 met 1.25 glip
	10:20 am	87 u P							
	12:00 pm	p 119 u							500 Met
	5:30 pm	p 101 u							
	9:35 pm	109 u							
11/16/05 Wed	7:30 am	p 94 u							500 Met 1.25 Glip
	10:15 am	92 u P							
	12:00 pm	p 101 u							
	3:50 pm	115 u							500 Met
	5:45 pm	p 105 u							
	8:35 pm	111 u P							
11/17/05 Thu	8:20 am	p 100 u							500 Met 1.25 Glip
	12:10 pm	p 114 u							
	5:30 pm	85 u P							500 Met
	8:15 pm	100 u P							
	11:05 pm	104 u							
11/18/05 Fri	8:00 am	100 u							500 met 1.25 glip
	10:30 am	94 u P							
	11:55 am	p 94 u							
	4:00 pm	p 95 u							500 Met

Date	Time	Glucose	0	40	65	130	180	601	Comment
11/18/05 Fri	9:45 pm	118 u P							Myrna's BD Party
11/19/05 Sat	8:00 am	p 120 u							Too Muxh Intake Last Night/Party
	8:00 am	E -							500 Met 1.25 Glip
	12:15 pm	p 112 u							
	6:00 pm	p 95 u							500 met
	8:35 pm	p 104 u P							
	10:00 pm	E - IS							
	11:00 pm	103 uc							Migraine @ 10:00 PM. BP High?
11/20/05 Sun	8:00 am	p 93 u							Migraine @ 10:00 PM 1 Hour
	8:44 am	100 uc							500 Met 1.25 Glip
	9:45 am	65 u P							WT @ 209.4-Lowest Yet!
	12:25 pm	p 101 u							
	6:15 pm	p 115 u							PA Blair Ridge - 500 Met
	11:35 pm	109 u							PA Blair Ridge
11/21/05 Mon	8:30 am	p 105 u							500 Met 1.25 Glip
	11:10 am	p 110 u							Forgot to Eat Breakfast
	4:00 pm	p 99 u							Late Lunch
	7:00 pm	E -							Public Appearance-Miller's Merry Ma
	8:30 pm	p 117 u							Forgot Medine @ 5:00 pM
	9:10 pm	E -							Late Supper
	11:30 pm	116 u P							
11/22/05 Tue	8:20 am	p 113 u							500 Met 1.25 Glip
	9:40 am	68 u P							Usually see a drop at this time
11/23/05 Wed	6:45 am	p 112 u							
	9:25 am	74 u P							
	12:15 pm	p 103 u							
	4:35 pm	p 96 u							500 Met
	9:05 pm	116 u P							
11/24/05 Thu	8:30 am	p 110 u							
	12:30 pm	p 112 u							500 met 1.25 glip
	5:05 pm	p 125 u							500 Met

161

Date	Time	Glucose	0	40	65	130	180	601	Comment
11/24/05 Thu	10:00 pm	138 uc							1.25 Glip - Thanksgiving Intake!
11/25/05 Fri	6:15 am	p 111 u							500 Met 1.25 Glip
	11:30 am	p 118 u							Have A Cold
	4:30 pm	p 109 u							500 Met
	11:15 pm	126 u							Ate Diet Apple Pie-Fish
11/26/05 Sat	8:15 am	p 109 u							500 Met 1.25 Glip
	12:00 pm	p 98 u							
	5:45 pm	p 138 u							500 Met
	11:00 pm	140 uc							1.25 Glip
11/27/05 Sun	8:00 am	p 109 u							500 Met 1.25 Glip 208.2 Lbs
	12:30 pm	p 115 u							PA Gilead
	9:00 pm	154 uc							Late Meds 500 Met 1.25 Glip
11/28/05 Mon	7:50 am	p 114 u							500 Mey 1.25 Glip 208.6 Lbs
	12:35 pm	p 114 u							
	3:35 pm	103 u							
	6:35 pm	p 121 uc							
	11:35 pm	89 u							500 Met 1.25 Glip
11/29/05 Tue	8:30 am	p 109 u							On Track
	12:20 pm	p 112 u							500 Met 1.25 Glip
	5:15 pm	104 uc							
	8:00 pm	87 u P							500 Met 1.25 Glip
11/30/05 Wed	8:25 am	p 104 u							500 Met 1.25 Glip
	12:05 pm	p 107 u							
	4:00 pm	p 111 u							500 Met 1.25 Glip
	9:30 pm	99 u							
12/01/05 Thu	7:05 am	E - S							Weight @ 205.8 lbs !
	7:15 am	p 107 u							500 Met 1.25 Glip
	11:40 am	p 115 u							
	5:00 pm	p 103 u							
	7:00 pm	E - S							
	9:00 pm	105 u P							500 Met 1.25 Glip

Date	Time	Glucose	0	40	65	130	180	601	Comment
12/02/05 Fri	8:05 am	p 61 u							500Met 1.25 Glip
	12:00 pm	p 100 u							
12/03/05 Sat	5:20 pm	p 100 u							500 met 1.25 glip
	8:00 am	p 107 u							500 met 1.25 glip
	10:30 am	93 u P							
	12:00 pm	p 102 u							500 met 1.25 glip
	4:45 pm	92 u							
	6:20 pm	p 82 u							
12/04/05 Sun	8:00 am	p 115 u							500 met 1.25 glip ate late
	9:00 pm	p 79 u							500 met 1.25 glip
12/05/05 Mon	8:00 am	p 123 u							
	12:00 pm	p 106 u							500 met 1.25 glip
	5:00 pm	p 101 u							
	8:00 pm	125 u P							500 met 1.25 glip
12/06/05 Tue	8:00 am	p 130 u							
	11:50 am	p 114 u							500 met 1.25 glip
	6:20 pm	p 83 u							
12/07/05 Wed	8:00 am	p 102 u							500 met 1.25 glip
	11:50 am	p 91 u							500 met 1.25 glip
	4:35 pm	p 100 u							
	8:10 pm	85 u P							500 met 1.25 glip
	11:00 pm	77 u P							great-chicken and rice combo great
12/08/05 Thu	7:20 am	p 96 uc							500 met 1.25 glip-Lab Fast
	10:00 am	85 uc							Fasting For LABWORK
	3:30 pm	p 93 u							
	9:05 pm	106 u							
12/09/05 Fri	8:30 am	p 119 u							500 Met 1.25 Glip
	12:20 pm	p 92 u							
	4:45 pm	p 108 u							500 Met 1.25 Glip
	9:50 pm	113 u							
12/10/05 Sat	8:25 am	p 115 u							500 Met 1.25 Glip

163

Date	Time	Glucose	0	40	65	130	180	601	Comment
12/10/05 Sat	12:20 pm	p 111 u							500 Met 1.25 Glip
	4:40 pm	p 125 u							500 Met 1.25 Glip
12/11/05 Sun	9:00 am	p 106 u							
	12:30 pm	p 102 u							Late Dinner-Public Ap Dukes
	7:30 pm	p 90 u							500 Met 1.25 Glip
12/12/05 Mon	7:30 am	p 115 u							
	11:40 am	p 102 u							
	3:00 pm	p 110 u P							
	5:00 pm	p 101 u							500 Met 1.25 Glip
	8:50 pm	108 u							
12/13/05 Tue	7:00 am	p 107 u							500 Met 1.25 Glip
	11:30 am	p 107 u							
	4:00 pm	p 120 u							500 Met 1.25 Glip
	6:05 pm	p 108 u							Need To eat smaller servings
	9:45 pm	114 u							500 Met 1.25 Glip
12/14/05 Wed	5:45 am	p 108 u							
	7:50 am	83 u							
	12:35 pm	p 99 u							500 Met 1.25 Glip
	4:15 pm	p 97 u							
	7:30 pm	66 u P							500 Met 1.25 Glip
12/15/05 Thu	8:30 am	p 119 u							
	11:50 am	p 107 u							Ate Late Lunch-No Meter Available
	1:40 pm	E -							500 Met 1.25 Glip
	5:20 pm	100 u							Excellent
	7:30 pm	77 u P							500 Met 1.25 Glip
12/16/05 Fri	7:50 am	p 106 u							
	8:30 am	p 118 u							
	11:05 am	101 u							
	12:15 pm	p 102 u							
	5:00 pm	p 111 u							500 Met 1.25 Glip
	8:30 pm	95 u P							

Date	Time	Glucose	0	40	65	130	180	601	Comment
12/17/05 Sat	8:30 am	p 95 u							500 Met 1.25 Glip
	12:40 pm	p 102 u							500 met 1.25 glip
	5:00 pm	p 91 u							
	8:10 pm	89 u P							500 met 1.25 glilp
12/18/05 Sun	8:15 am	p 114 u							
	12:10 pm	p 107 u							
	4:20 pm	p 97 u							500 Met 1.25 Glip PA Did Not Eat Late Meal
	9:15 pm	p 94 u							500 Met 1.25 Glip 204.6 lbs
12/19/05 Mon	8:15 am	p 117 u							
	12:40 pm	p 100 u							
	4:10 pm	p 111 u							500 met 1.25 glip
	5:30 pm	p 107 u							
	10:20 pm	95 u							
12/20/05 Tue	7:15 am	p 93 u							500 Met 1.25 Glip
	12:25 pm	p 106 u							
	4:30 pm	p 92 u							500 Met 1.25 Glip
	8:45 pm	86 u							
12/21/05 Wed	6:50 am	p 97 u							500 Met 1.25 Glip
	6:25 pm	p 98 u							500 met 1.25 glip
	7:30 pm	82 u P							Ate Cherries & Raisin Cookies
12/22/05 Thu	7:30 am	p 118 u							500 Met 1.25 Glip-Cold
	3:50 pm	p 105 u							500 Met 1.25 Glip
12/23/05 Fri	9:15 am	p 94 u							500 Met 1.25 Glip
	1:00 pm	102 u							
	6:00 pm	p 80 u							500 Met 1.25 Glip
	8:10 pm	87 u P							
12/24/05 Sat	6:00 am	p 123 u							500 Met 1.25 Glip
	10:20 am	99 u							
	12:25 pm	p 115 u							500 Met 1.25 lip
12/25/05 Sun	3:15 pm	p 115 u							500 Met 1.25 Glip
	9:15 am	p 122 u							

Date	Time	Glucose	0	40	65	130	180	601	Comment
12/25/05 Sun	11:45 am	p 108 u							Cold
	3:15 pm	173 u P							
	5:50 pm	p 123 u							500 Met 1.25 Glip
12/26/05 Mon	8:45 am	p 130 u							500 Met 1.25 Glip
	12:05 pm	p 107 u							
	3:20 pm	100 u P							
	5:00 pm	p 90 u							500 Met 1.25 Glip
	8:20 pm	93 u P							
12/27/05 Tue	9:40 am	p 122 u							500 Met 1.25 Glip
	12:50 pm	p 120 u							Cold
	5:00 pm	p 85 u							500 Met 1.25 Glip
	9:00 pm	90 u							
12/28/05 Wed	7:00 am	p 108 u							500 Met 1.25 Glip
	4:00 pm	p 122 u							500 Met 1.25 Glip
	5:55 pm	65 uc P							May have to reduce Glip
	6:30 pm	E - S							Ate Banana-Raisins-Glucose Tab
12/29/05 Thu	8:25 am	p 131 u							500 Met 1.25 Glip
	11:30 am	p 110 u							Cold
	4:10 pm	84 uc P							500 Met-No Glip!
	7:20 pm	97 u P							
12/30/05 Fri	7:50 am	p 103 u							500 Met 1.25 Glip-Slight Cold
	12:00 pm	95 u							
	5:55 pm	p 79 u							500 met
	7:30 pm	86 u P							
12/31/05 Sat	8:30 am	p 98 u							500 met 1.25 glip
	12:00 pm	p 102 u							
	2:35 pm	130 u P							
	5:00 pm	p 108 u							500 met
	7:40 pm	112 u P							New Years Eve Party
	9:30 pm	E - S P							Special Food/Mary/Party
	10:45 pm	E - S P							Special Food/Mary/Party

Date	Time	Glucose	Comment
01/01/06 Sun	9:00 am	p 123 u	500 Met 1.25 Glip Happy NY!
	1:05 pm	p 104 u	
	4:00 pm	p 118 u	Happy NY 500 Met
01/02/06 Mon	8:00 am	p 114 u	500 Met 1.25 Glip
	12:30 pm	p 105 u	
	4:50 pm	p 100 u	500 Met
	8:20 pm	122 u P	
01/03/06 Tue	9:00 am	p 114 u	500 Met 1.25 Glip Happy NY
	10:25 am	E - DS	Holiday Over-Eating-Back On Track
	10:30 am	E - ES	Not Exercising-To Begin 1 4 05
	10:55 am	90 u P	
01/04/06 Wed	5:00 pm	p 105 u	500 Met
	9:30 am	p 96 u	500 Met 1.25 Glip
	1:00 pm	p 94 u	
	5:20 pm	p 92 u	500 Met
	8:40 pm	116 u P	
01/05/06 Thu	8:30 am	p 113 u	500 Met 1.25 Glip
	10:50 am	84 u P	
	12:10 pm	p 95 u	
	2:00 pm	E - ES	First Day at gym/B Ball
	4:15 pm	p 95 u	
	5:20 pm	p 91 u	500 Met
01/06/06 Fri	8:15 pm	83 uc P	!st Day Back At Gym
	8:15 am	p 110 u	500 Met 1.25 Glip
	11:50 am	p 92 u	
	4:40 pm	p 90 u	500 Met
	8:40 pm	143 u P	Ate at 5:30 Had Banana/Beans/Rice
01/07/06 Sat	8:40 am	p 111 u	500 Met 1.25 Glip
	12:15 pm	p 95 u	
	3:35 pm	p 68 u	500 Met
	8:55 pm	162 u	Very Likely Diet-Chinese Food

Date	Time	Glucose	0	40	65	130	180	601	Comment
01/08/06 Sun	8:45 am	p 126 u							500 Met 1.25 Glip
	12:05 pm	p 94 u							
	3:55 pm	p 103 u							
	9:15 pm	p 105 u							
01/09/06 Mon	8:50 am	p 98 u							500 Met PA
									Gilliad PA
	11:50 am	p 84 u							500 Met 1.25 Glip
	2:10 pm	E - ES							
	3:55 pm	p 91 u							Back @ Y-Basketball-2nd Day
	9:30 pm	p 88 u P							500 Met-InControl-Gym Exercise-Diet
01/10/06 Tue	7:35 am	p 97 u							500 Met 1.25 Glip
	12:15 pm	p 102 u							
	3:25 pm	101 u P							
	4:45 pm	p 107 u							
	9:05 pm	p 94 uc							500 Met
01/11/06 Wed	8:45 am	p 103 u							Day 3 at Gym
	12:15 pm	p 73 u							500 Met 1.25 Glip
	3:45 pm	97 uc							
	5:10 pm	p 90 u							Gym at 1 Hour
	8:25 pm	p 95 u							500 Met
01/12/06 Thu	8:30 am	p 94 u							500 Met 1.25 Glip
	12:20 pm	p 86 u							
	5:25 pm	p 83 u							
	8:55 pm	p 144 uc							Forgot To Take Metformin
									500 Met-forgot to take @ 5:00
01/13/06 Fri	8:05 am	p 103 u							500 Met
	12:10 pm	p 103 u							Gym Workout @ 11:45 AM
	5:10 pm	p 88 u							500 Met
	9:20 pm	p 89 u							
01/14/06 Sat	8:10 am	p 93 u							500 Met 1.25 Glip
	12:15 pm	p 101 u							
	5:00 pm	p 100 u							500 Met
01/15/06 Sun	9:05 am	p 102 u							500 Met 1.25 Glip

Date	Time	Glucose	Comment
01/15/06 Sun	12:20 pm	p 85 u	500 Met-Pie & Cake/BD Ashley
	6:15 pm	p 110 u	500 met 1.25 Glip
01/16/06 Mon	8:15 am	p 105 u	Heavy Workout 1 Hr 20 Min-Gym
	11:45 am	p 99 uc	500 Met @ 5:00 PM
	4:10 pm	p 97 u	Meal Sizes Need to Be Reduced
	8:30 pm	148 u P	500 Met 1.25 Glip
01/17/06 Tue	8:20 am	p 102 u	Weight Trends Elevating 204-212 lbs
	8:20 am	E - DS	Start Focusing On Smaller Lunch
	9:30 am	E - DS	Start Focusing On smaller Dinners
	9:32 am	E - DS	
	12:15 pm	p 90 u	
	3:25 pm	81 u P	500 Met
	5:05 pm	p 91 u	Prepare to Eliminate Glipizide
	6:50 pm	E - S	
	7:55 pm	p 95 u	
01/18/06 Wed	7:50 pm	p 100 u	500 Met 1.25 Glip
	12:05 pm	p 76 u	
	4:40 pm	p 76 u	
	8:30 pm	p 129 u	500 Met
01/19/06 Thu	8:00 am	p 100 u	Bible Study 6:30-7:45P
	12:00 pm	p 113 u	500 Met 1.25 Glip
	5:00 pm	p 100 u	
	9:00 pm	p 93 u	500 Met
01/20/06 Fri	8:00 am	p 99 u	Continue Small Meals
	12:35 pm	p 106 u	1.25 Glip 500 Met
	4:40 pm	p 84 u	
	8:20 pm	E - S P	Took 500 met Late-Forgot @ 5:00 PM
01/21/06 Sat	9:20 pm	p 97 u	
	8:20 am	p 102 u	500 met 1.25 glip
	12:05 pm	p 83 u	
	5:00 pm	p 90 u	500 met

Chart axis values: 0   40   65   130   180   601

Date	Time	Glucose	0	40	65	130	180	601	Comment
01/21/06 Sat	7:45 pm	p 131 u				■			Ate Large Dinner / Siding
	8:00 pm	E - P							Banana/Raspberries/Nuts/PB
01/22/06 Sun	8:30 am	p 100 u				■			500 Met 1.25 Glip
	12:15 pm	p 92 u			■				
	4:10 pm	p 78 u			■				500 Met
	9:05 pm	p 95 u			■				PA-Gilliad
01/23/06 Mon	6:30 am	p 111 u				■			500 Met 1.25 Glip
	12:00 pm	p 121 u				■			
	4:30 pm	p 87 u			■				500 Met
01/24/06 Tue	8:00 am	E - S							Meter Failure-Used Ultima
	8:30 am	p 96 u			■				500 Met 1.25 Glip-Ultima
	12:00 pm	p 100 u			■				
	4:50 pm	E - S							Back On Elite
	5:00 pm	p 112 u				■			500 Met 1.25 Glip
	9:00 pm	p 132 u				■			
01/25/06 Wed	9:00 am	p 106 u				■			500 Met 1.25 Glip
	12:30 pm	p 95 u			■				
	3:15 pm	103 uc P				■			Accu-Check On Line-New
	5:15 pm	p 80 u			■				500 Met 1.25 Glip
	8:00 pm	p 97 u			■				
01/26/06 Thu	8:30 am	p 103 u				■			500 Met 1.25 Glip
	10:10 am	74 u P			■				Consider Eliminating Glipizide
	1:00 pm	p 109 u				■			
	4:30 pm	p 95 u			■				500 Met
	9:45 pm	p 89 u			■				Council Meeting-Unnessary Stress
01/27/06 Fri	8:30 am	p 88 u			■				500 Met 1.25 Glip
	4:35 pm	p 104 u				■			500 Met
	8:45 pm	109 u				■			Stressful Day-Hilda In Hosp
01/28/06 Sat	8:30 am	p 117 u				■			500 Mdet 1.25 Glip
	12:05 pm	p 122 u				■			Stress Related
	5:15 pm	p 105 uc				■			500 Met-Stress Related

Date	Time	Glucose	0	40	65	130	180	601	Comment
01/29/06 Sun	7:40 am	p 94 u							500 Met 1325 Glip
	12:05 pm	p 168 uc							Stress-NJ@ PAs & Thurs Meeting
	4:25 pm	p 119 u							500 Met
	9:10 pm	p 102 u							Returned From Gilead
01/30/06 Mon	8:20 am	p 114 u							500 Met 1.25 Glip
	12:20 pm	p 108 u							
	5:10 pm	p 93 u							500 met
	10:05 pm	p 125 u							IceCream/Berries
01/31/06 Tue	8:00 am	p 107 u							500 Met 1.25 Glip
	12:00 pm	p 120 uc							Scheduled Meeting/One/Stress
	3:00 pm	p 106 u							
	3:30 pm	E - DS							Early Dinner
	6:00 pm	E - S							500 Met
	7:00 pm	p 86 u							
02/01/06 Wed	8:00 am	p 104 u							500 Met 1.25 Glip
	12:00 pm	p 133 u							Intense Exercise
	4:25 pm	p 109 u							500 Met
	8:10 pm	p 85 u							
02/02/06 Thu	7:35 am	113 u							500 Met 1.25 Glip
	8:35 am	p 98 u							
	12:05 pm	p 88 u							
	4:30 pm	p 79 u							
	5:45 pm	E - S P							500 Met-forgot at dinner time
02/03/06 Fri	8:30 pm	p 114 u							500 Met 1.25 Glip
	7:35 am	p 118 u							
	12:00 pm	p 109 u							500 Met
	4:50 pm	p 92 u							500 Met 2 Glim
02/04/06 Sat	7:35 am	p 112 u							
	12:00 pm	p 111 u							500 Met-Ate late
	3:45 pm	p 97 u							
	5:15 pm	p 100 u							

Date	Time	Glucose	0	40	65	130	180	601	Comment
02/05/06 Sun	8:10 am	p 109 u							500 Met 1.25 Glip
	12:05 pm	p 108 u							
	4:00 pm	p 100 u							
02/06/06 Mon	8:15 am	p 112 u							500 Met
	11:30 am	p 82 u							500 Met 1.25 Glip
	4:30 pm	p 86 u							
02/07/06 Tue	8:25 am	p 97 u							500 Met
	11:55 am	p 99 u							500 Met 1.25 Glip
	4:15 pm	p 95 u							
02/08/06 Wed	8:00 am	p 104 u							500 Met
	12:00 pm	p 100 u							500 Met 1.25 Glip Plugged Reading
	5:30 pm	p 86 u							500 Met
02/09/06 Thu	7:50 am	p 91 u							500 Met 1.25 Glip
	12:40 pm	p 90 u							
	4:50 pm	p 82 u							500 Met 1.25 Glip
02/10/06 Fri	8:15 am	p 111 u							
	12:30 pm	p 90 u							500 Met
	5:00 pm	p 80 u							
	10:00 pm	p 80 u							500 Met
02/11/06 Sat	8:40 am	p 97 u							500 Met 1.25 Glip
	12:30 pm	87 u							
	4:15 pm	p 105 u							500 Met
02/12/06 Sun	8:30 am	p 101 u							
	8:35 am	p 104 u							500 met 1.25 glip
	12:10 pm	p 100 u							
	4:35 pm	p 94 u							500 Met
02/13/06 Mon	7:55 pm	p 104 u							
	8:15 am	p 113 u							500 Met 1.25 Glip
	11:45 am	p 97 u							500 Met
	4:45 pm	p 81 u							
	8:00 pm	p 89 u							500 Met Need to Reduce this meal by 50%

Date	Time	Glucose	0	40	65	130	180	601	Comment
02/14/06 Tue	8:00 am	p 100 u							500 Met 1.25 Glip
	12:10 pm	p 95 u							
	4:40 pm	p 84 u							500 Met
	9:10 pm	p 88 u							
02/15/06 Wed	7:45 am	p 90 u							500 Met 1.25 Glip 204.8 lbs
	9:00 am	p 96 u							Late Breakfast
	11:55 am	p 91 u							
	5:15 pm	p 81 u							500 Met
	9:15 pm	p 95 u							Under 100 entire Day
02/16/06 Thu	8:15 am	p 96 u							500 Met 1.25 Glip 204.6 LBS
	12:00 pm	p 82 u							
	4:35 pm	p 89 u							500 met
	9:00 pm	p 90 u							
02/17/06 Fri	8:05 am	p 99 u							500 Met 1.25 Glip
	12:00 pm	p 87 u							
	4:35 pm	p 80 u							500 Met
	9:15 pm	p 130 u							Huge 12" Seafood Sub for Dinner
02/18/06 Sat	7:35 am	p 120 u							500 Met 1.25 Glip
	12:15 pm	p 91 u							Back on track
	4:45 pm	p 92 u							500 met
	9:05 pm	p 105 u							
02/19/06 Sun	8:00 am	p 109 u							500 Met 1.25 Glip
	12:40 pm	p 91 u							
	4:25 pm	p 88 u							500 Met
	8:55 pm	p 106 u							Public Appearance
02/20/06 Mon	7:30 am	p 99 u							500 Met 1.25 Glip
	12:15 pm	p 94 u							
	4:30 pm	p 97 u							500 Met
	8:30 pm	p 102 u							
02/21/06 Tue	8:30 am	p 102 u							500 met 1.25 glip
	12:15 pm	p 101 u							

Date	Time	Glucose	0	40	65	130	180	601	Comment
02/21/06 Tue	5:05 pm	p 87 u							500 Met
	10:30 pm	p 95 u							
02/22/06 Wed	8:05 am	p 98 u							500 Met 1.25 Glip
	12:15 pm	p 95 u							Estimate-did not record
	5:05 pm	p 90 u							500 Met
	9:10 pm	p 92 u							Last Two weeks - Fantastic Control
02/23/06 Thu	8:00 am	p 100 u							500 Met 1.25 Glip
	12:00 pm	p 95 u							
	4:30 pm	p 91 u							500 Met
	8:45 pm	p 113 u							Anniversary Dinner/Bread
02/24/06 Fri	8:00 am	p 112 u							500 Met 1.25 Glip
	12:00 pm	p 98 u							
	6:00 pm	p 114 u							500 Met-Velma's Strawberry Pie
	10:00 pm	p 96 u							Back To Normal
02/25/06 Sat	8:20 am	p 102 u							500 Met 1.25 Glip
	12:10 pm	p 92 u							
	4:45 pm	p 72 u							500 Met
	9:15 pm	p 88 u							
02/26/06 Sun	8:20 am	p 103 u							500 Met 1.25 Glip
	12:00 pm	p 93 u							
	4:25 pm	p 88 u							500 Met
	9:00 pm	p 99 u							PA Gilead
02/27/06 Mon	7:50 am	p 105 u							500 Met 1.25 Glip
	11:50 am	p 93 u							
	4:10 pm	p 86 u							Forgot to take Metformin @ 4:10 PM
	8:15 pm	E - S P							Took 500 Metformin @ 8:15 PM
	9:02 pm	p 102 u							Forgot Metformin @ Dinner
02/28/06 Tue	7:10 am	p 94 u							500 Met 1.25 Glip
	11:55 am	p 105 u							
	4:50 pm	p 91 u							500 Met
	8:45 pm	p 83 u							

174

Date	Time	Glucose	0	40	65	130	180	601	Comment
03/01/06 Wed	7:15 am	p 96 u							500 Met 1.25 Glip
	12:05 pm	p 110 u							
	5:05 pm	p 100 u							
	8:15 pm	p 111 u							Met-Estimated reading/no meter
									Higher than normal
03/02/06 Thu	7:40 am	p 114 u							500 Met 1.25 Glip 204.4 lbs
	12:00 pm	p 98 u							
	4:00 pm	p E - DS							500 Met-Early Med/Lion Dnr Activity
									Late Meal Early Medicine
	6:25 pm	p 65 u							Less than 2.5 Hrs from Meal
	8:55 pm	116 u P							No Med Until 7:00 PM-ProSlot Work
03/03/06 Fri	6:00 am	p 115 u							500 Met 1.25 Glip
	7:00 am	p E -							199.2 LBS-Record Low
	8:30 am	p 90 u							
	12:25 pm	p 95 u							
	5:00 pm	p 94 u							500 Met
	5:30 pm	E - S							Special Med @ 5:30 PM
	8:40 pm	p 102 u							
03/04/06 Sat	7:10 am	p 110 u							500 Met 1.25 Glip
	12:00 pm	p 113 u							
	4:25 pm	p 98 u							
	5:45 pm	E - S							
	9:15 pm	p 107 u							OOps -Forgot Metformin
									Late with 500 Met/forgot Took-5:45P
03/05/06 Sun	7:50 am	p 113 u							500 Met 1.25 Glip
	12:00 pm	p 125 u							Meter was cold-may have read high
	12:45 pm	p E - D							Ioretta's Birthday Luncheon
	5:05 pm	131 u							500 Met Ate Way too much @ Lunch
	8:25 pm	p 118 u							Still a little high from lunch
03/06/06 Mon	7:25 am	p 117 u							500 Met 1.25 Glip
	12:15 pm	p 87 u							Back on Track
	5:00 pm	p 94 u							500 Met
	9:15 pm	p 109 u							Need to back this meal down a bit
03/07/06 Tue	7:45 am	p 110 u							500 Met 1.25 Glip

Date	Time	Glucose	0	40	65	130	180	601	Comment
03/07/06 Tue	12:05 pm	p 94 u							500 Met
	5:00 pm	p 82 u							
	9:00 pm	p 96 u							
03/08/06 Wed	8:15 am	p 102 u							500 Met 1.25 Glip
	12:30 pm	p 90 u							
	4:45 pm	p 88 u							500 Met
	9:45 pm	p 102 u							
03/09/06 Thu	7:55 am	p 94 u							500 Met 1.25 Glip
	12:45 pm	p 89 u							
	5:00 pm	p 85 u							500 Met-Huge Dinner Tonite
03/10/06 Fri	8:15 am	p 112 u							500 Met 1.25 Glip-Ate Bread/Supper
	1:15 pm	p 114 u							1/2 Fish Sandwich
	5:25 pm	p 101 u							500 Met Large Dinner & Wheat Buns
	8:50 pm	p 110 u							
03/11/06 Sat	7:20 am	p 117 u							500 Met 1.25 Glip
	12:45 pm	p 100 u							
	4:40 pm	p 94 u							500 Met
	8:10 pm	p 100 u							
03/12/06 Sun	8:35 am	p 121 u							500 Met 1.25 Pizza Last Night
	9:55 am	71 u P							
	12:00 pm	p 118 u							Church
	4:25 pm	p 106 u							500 Met
	9:10 pm	p 106 u							PA Gilead
03/13/06 Mon	5:25 am	p 104 u							
	8:00 am	p E - DS							Ate Breakfast 500 Met 1.25 Glip
	12:00 pm	p 97 u							
	4:00 pm	p 99 u							500 Met
	9:25 pm	p 102 u							Beans & Nuts-Rehearsal
03/14/06 Tue	7:55 am	p 112 u							500 Met 1.25 Glip
	12:36 pm	p 107 u							
	5:00 pm	p 93 u							500 Met

Date	Time	Glucose	Comment
03/14/06 Tue	8:55 pm	p 99 u	500 Met 1.25 Glip
03/15/06 Wed	6:55 am	p 104 u	Joe E's Brother's Funeral
	12:05 pm	p 104 u	500 Met forgot @ mealtime
	5:45 pm	E - S P	
	9:30 pm	p 102 u	
03/16/06 Thu	8:15 am	p 102 u	500 Met 1.25 Glip
	12:10 pm	p 96 u	
	4:55 pm	p 104 u	500 Mert
	9:15 pm	p 114 u	
03/17/06 Fri	7:35 am	p 105 u	500 Met 1.25 Glip
	12:05 pm	p 102 u	
	4:10 pm	p 96 u	500 Met
	9:55 pm	p 114 u	
03/18/06 Sat	8:00 am	p 107 u	500 Met 1.25 Glip
	12:30 pm	p 96 u	
	4:55 pm	p 87 u	500 Met
	9:30 pm	p 157 u	Pizza @ Din & Ron To Hospital
03/19/06 Sun	7:55 am	p 107 u	500 Met 1.25 Glip
	12:05 pm	p 111 u	Church/Ron In Hospital
	5:15 pm	E - DST	500 Met @ Lutheran/Ron
	9:35 pm	p 100 u	Good recovery
03/20/06 Mon	8:40 am	p 91 u	500 Met 1.25 Glip
	4:45 pm	p 94 u	500 Met
	9:00 pm	p 96 u	
03/21/06 Tue	8:40 am	p 103 u	500 Met 1.25 Glip
	12:00 pm	p 93 u	
	4:35 pm	p 100 u	500 Met
	9:45 pm	p 94 u	
03/22/06 Wed	7:05 am	p 90 u	500 Met 1.25 Glip
	5:50 pm	p 92 u	500 Met
	9:30 pm	p 150 u	Ron' Surg/Mexican Food/White Flour

Date	Time	Glucose	0	40	65	130	180	601	Comment
03/23/06 Thu	7:50 am	p 105 u							500 Met 1.25 Glip
	12:25 pm	p 95 u							500 Met
	4:30 pm	p 79 u							
	9:20 pm	p 90 u							
03/24/06 Fri	8:05 am	p 95 u							500 Met 1.25 Glip
	12:25 pm	p 86 u							
	5:00 pm	p 107 u							Forgot 500 Metformin
	9:10 pm	p 111 u							
03/25/06 Sat	8:00 am	p 118 u							500 Met 1.25 Glip
	12:20 pm	p 97 u							
	4:40 pm	p 96 u							500 Met
	8:40 pm	p 102 u							
03/26/06 Sun	7:50 am	p 116 u							500 Met 1.25 Glip
	12:20 pm	p 118 u							Church
	4:30 pm	p 105 u							500 Met
	8:50 pm	p 105 u							
03/27/06 Mon	7:55 am	p 107 u							500 Met 1.25 Glip
	12:20 pm	p 99 u							
	4:30 pm	p 92 u							500 Met
	8:20 pm	p 95 u							
03/28/06 Tue	5:10 am	p 99 u							To Early For Medication
	8:10 am	p 117 u							500 Met 1.25 Glip
	12:00 pm	p 90 u							
	5:00 pm	p 98 u							500 Met
03/29/06 Wed	8:15 am	p 101 u							500 Met 1.25 Glip
	5:00 pm	p 96 u							
	8:35 pm	p 111 u							Forgot Metfomin-Ron Went Home
03/30/06 Thu	7:20 am	p 103 u							500 Met 1.25 Glip
	1:20 pm	p 123 u							Ramp Gilead Prep
	5:25 pm	p 93 u							500 Met-Cookie visited
03/31/06 Fri	7:05 am	p 121 u							500 Met 1.25 Glip

178

Date	Time	Glucose	Comment
03/31/06 Fri	6:10 pm	p 98 u	500 Met
	9:05 pm	p 120 u	
04/01/06 Sat	6:45 am	p 110 u	500 Met 1.25 Glip
	5:00 pm	p E -	500 Met
04/02/06 Sun	5:00 am	p 97 u	500 Met 1.25 Glip
	1:20 pm	100 u	
	5:00 pm	p 126 u	500 Met
	9:45 pm	p 116 u	
04/03/06 Mon	6:55 am	p 115 u	500 Met 1.25 Glip
	12:00 pm	p 105 u	
	5:00 pm	100 u	500 Met
	9:45 pm	p 107 u	
04/04/06 Tue	7:45 am	p 125 u	500 Met 1.25 Glip
	4:15 pm	p 132 u	500 Met
	7:25 pm	p 119 u	
04/05/06 Wed	7:30 am	p 114 u	500 Met 1.25 Glip
	12:25 pm	p 112 u	
	4:55 pm	p 102 u	
	8:25 pm	p 108 u	500 Met
04/06/06 Thu	6:20 am	p 107 u	500 Met 1.25 Glip
	5:30 pm	p 98 u	500 Met
04/07/06 Fri	7:55 am	p 102 u	500 Met 1.25 Glip
	6:20 pm	p 95 u	500 Met
04/08/06 Sat	7:10 am	p 117 u	500 Met 1.25 Glip
	5:30 pm	p 111 u	500 Met
04/09/06 Sun	6:31 am	p 119 u	500 Met 1.25 Glip
	4:20 pm	p 100 u	500 Met
04/10/06 Mon	7:30 am	p 109 u	500 Met 1.25 Glip
	3:30 pm	E - E	Major work-out + Gilead
	6:20 pm	p 109 u	500 Met
04/11/06 Tue	7:35 am	p 111 u	500 Met 1.25 Glip

Graph axis values: 0, 40, 65, 130, 180, 601

Date	Time	Glucose	0	40	65	130	180	601	Comment
04/11/06 Tue	2:05 pm	p 99 u							Late Lunch–Gilead
	4:10 pm	p 94 u							
	5:00 pm	p E -							
04/12/06 Wed	7:40 am	p 109 u							500 Met
	12:20 pm	E - DS							500 Met 1.25 Glip
									Drank too much Coffee during day!
	4:00 pm	E - ISTY							Migraine-40 Minutes - 4:00 PM
	4:55 pm	p 83 u							500 Met
	5:00 pm	p E -							
04/13/06 Thu	7:15 am	p 95 u							500 Met 1.25 Glip
	4:00 pm	E - D							Major Coffee Intake Reduction
	5:00 pm	p E -							500 Met
	5:10 pm	p 108 u							
04/14/06 Fri	5:00 am	p 102 u							500 Met 1.25 Glip
	2:30 pm	p 94 u							Late Lunch
	5:00 pm	p E -							
	8:20 pm	p 92 u							500 Met-Late Dinner
04/15/06 Sat	8:15 am	p 105 u							500 Met 1.25 Glip
	5:00 pm	p E -							500 Met
04/16/06 Sun	8:20 am	p 109 u							500 Met 1.25 Glip
	5:00 pm	p E -							
	8:20 pm	p 125 u							500 Met -Late Med/Gilead
04/17/06 Mon	6:55 am	p 90 u							500 Met 1.25 Glip
	5:00 pm	p E -							500 Met
	6:05 pm	p 87 u							
04/18/06 Tue	7:05 am	p 101 u							500 Met 1.25 Glip
	4:35 pm	p 92 u							500 Met
	5:00 pm	p E -							500 Met
04/19/06 Wed	7:25 am	p 95 u							500 Met 1.25 Glip
	4:50 pm	91 u							500 Met
	5:00 pm	p E -							
04/20/06 Thu	7:40 am	p 94 u							500 Met 1.25 Glip

Date	Time	Glucose	0	40	65	130	180	601	Comment
04/20/06 Thu	5:00 pm	p E -							500 Met
04/21/06 Fri	7:00 am	p 96 u							500 Met 1.25 Glip
	5:00 pm	p E -							500 Met
04/22/06 Sat	6:25 am	p 109 u							500 Met 1.25 Glip
	5:00 pm	p E -							500 Met
04/23/06 Sun	8:15 am	p 106 u							500 Met 1.25 Glip
	5:10 pm	88 u							500 Met
04/24/06 Mon	7:25 am	p 103 u							500 Met 1.25 Glip
	4:20 pm	93 u							500 Met
04/25/06 Tue	8:00 am	p 97 u							500 Met 1.25 Glip
	12:15 pm	p 96 u							
	5:15 pm	p E -							
04/26/06 Wed	7:50 am	p 94 u							500 Met
	5:00 pm	p 100 u							500 Met 1.25 Glip
04/27/06 Thu	7:20 am	p 113 u							500 Met
	4:40 pm	p 96 u							500 Met
04/28/06 Fri	7:30 am	E - S							Lincoln Died
	7:45 am	p 98 u							500 Met 1.25 Glip
	5:40 pm	p 85 u							500 Met
04/29/06 Sat	5:25 am	p 128 u							500 Met 1.25 Glip
	5:25 am	p E - EST							Lion Breakfast
	11:55 am	p 110 u							
	5:25 pm	p 98 u							
04/30/06 Sun	8:35 am	p 103 u							500 Met
	12:30 pm	p 110 u							500 Met 1.25 Glip
	4:40 pm	p 79 u							Met Cold-ACCU CHECK-Guessed rdg
	8:55 pm	p 113 u							500 Met
05/01/06 Mon	8:20 am	p 106 u							Gilead NJ Program
	5:30 pm	p 88 u							500 Met 1.25 Glip
05/02/06 Tue	7:40 am	p 108 u							500 Met
	5:30 pm	p 91 u							500 Met 1.25 Glip
									500 Met

Date	Time	Glucose	0	40	65	130	180	601	Comment
05/03/06 Wed	7:40 am	p 96 u							500 Met 1.25 Glip
	11:00 am	E - T							Lincoln's Funeral
	5:20 pm	p 89 u							500 Met
05/04/06 Thu	7:35 am	p 98 u							500 Met
	5:10 pm	p E -							500 Met 1.25 Glip
05/05/06 Fri	7:05 am	p 101 u							
	5:10 pm	p 83 u							
	5:10 pm	p E -							500 Met
05/06/06 Sat	7:45 am	p 93 u							500 Met 1.25 Glip
	5:25 pm	p 89 u							500 Met
05/07/06 Sun	7:25 am	p 90 u							500 Met 1.25 Glip
	4:30 pm	p E - T							500 Met
	8:55 pm	p 122 u							Large Dinner/Gilead
05/08/06 Mon	8:00 am	p 96 u							500 Met 1.25 Glip
	5:55 pm	p 94 u							500 Met
05/09/06 Tue	7:25 am	p 90 u							500 Met 1.25 Glip
	8:00 pm	E - S P							Forgot 5:00 pm Met-Took @ 8:30 pm
05/10/06 Wed	7:30 am	p 110 u							500 Met 1.25 Glip
	5:00 pm	p E - S							500 Met
05/11/06 Thu	7:45 am	p 83 u							500 Met 1.25 Glip
	5:00 pm	E - S							500 Met
05/12/06 Fri	6:05 am	p 90 uc							500 Met No Glipizide!
	11:30 am	p 108 u							500 Met- Concern For Taking Extra
	5:25 pm	p 85 u							Berries & Eddy's
	9:10 pm	p 106 u							Ate Again-Two Lean Steaks-Bad!
	10:00 pm	E - DS							No Med Yet
05/13/06 Sat	4:30 am	108 u							500 Met No Glip
	8:00 am	p E - S							500 Met
	5:20 pm	p E - S							Alumni Gathering/North Miami/JTHS
	9:15 pm	p 93 u							500 Met No Glip
05/14/06 Sun	8:00 am	p E - S							

Date	Time	Glucose	Comment
05/14/06 Sun	8:25 am	p 93 u	500 Met-No Glip
	5:20 pm	104 u	Gilead-Did Not Eat-No Met
	9:15 pm	p 93 u	Late Dinner 500 Met
05/15/06 Mon	7:20 am	p 92 u	500 Met-No Glip
	5:20 pm	p 85 u	500 Met
	9:15 pm	p 101 u	
05/16/06 Tue	7:45 am	p 97 u	500 Met-No Glip
	12:10 pm	p 102 u	
	5:05 pm	p 89 u	500 Met
	9:15 pm	p 80 u	May Need To Reduce Metformin
05/17/06 Wed	7:35 am	p 97 u	500 Met-No lip
	5:25 pm	p 92 u	500 Met
05/18/06 Thu	7:10 am	p 90 u	500 Met
	5:25 pm	p 93 u	500 Met
	9:15 pm	p 89 u	
05/19/06 Fri	5:45 am	p 89 u	500 Met- Early Meds
	12:00 pm	p 97 u	
	6:15 pm	p 86 uc	250 Met & No Glipizide Again Today!
	9:15 pm	p 105 u	
05/20/06 Sat	6:45 am	p 100 u	500 Met
	11:45 am	p 109 u	
	5:50 pm	p 102 u	250 Met
	10:05 pm	p 99 u	
05/21/06 Sun	7:30 am	p 94 u	500 Met
	9:30 am	p E - DS	Ate Breakfast
	12:00 pm	p 114 u	250 Met
	4:10 pm	p 97 u	Super-No Glip and Reduced Metformin
	9:40 pm	p 97 u	500 Met
05/22/06 Mon	7:30 am	p 100 u	250 Met
	5:25 pm	p 75 u	
	9:15 pm	p 96 u	

Date	Time	Glucose	0	40	65	130	180	601	Comment
05/23/06 Tue	5:40 am	p 87 u							Looking Super
	4:35 pm	p 94 u							250 Met
	9:30 pm	p 90 u							Excellent!
05/24/06 Wed	5:10 am	p 90 u							
	8:30 am	p 110 u							500 Met-Late
	12:45 pm	p 102 u							
	5:05 pm	p 90 u							250 Met
	9:05 pm	p 90 u							
05/25/06 Thu	6:45 am	p 97 u							500 Met
	12:45 pm	p 104 u							
	4:30 pm	p 82 u							250 Met
	9:10 pm	p 88 u							Excellent
05/26/06 Fri	7:00 am	p 108 u							500 Met
	11:50 am	p 108 u							
	5:45 pm	p 93 u							250 Met
	10:45 pm	p 94 u							
05/27/06 Sat	5:00 am	p 94 u							
	8:00 am	p E -							
	5:00 pm	E -							
	9:25 pm	100 u							500 Met
05/28/06 Sun	8:30 am	p 91 u							250 Met
	4:30 pm	p E -							AccuCheck Meter
	8:40 pm	p 111 u							500 Met-AccuCheck-Amended
05/29/06 Mon	7:45 am	p 84 u							250 Met
	5:35 pm	p 88 u							AccuCheck Meter-Amended
	8:45 pm	p 90 u							500 Met-AccuCheck-Amended
05/30/06 Tue	7:40 am	p 89 u							250 Met
	4:45 pm	p 111 u							
	9:50 pm	p 94 u							500 Met
05/31/06 Wed	6:35 am	p 100 u							250 Met
	12:15 pm	p 116 u							500 Met

Date	Time	Glucose		0	40	65	130	180	601	Comment
05/31/06 Wed	5:05 pm	p 100 u								250 Met
	9:35 pm	p 100 u								
06/01/06 Thu	6:30 am	p 89 u								500 Met
	12:05 pm	p 109 u								
	5:25 pm	p 95 u								250 Met
	10:40 pm	p 97 u								
	5:30 am	p 88 u								
06/02/06 Fri	8:00 am	p E -								500 Met
	5:25 pm	p E -								250 Met
	9:55 pm	p 100 u								
06/03/06 Sat	7:50 am	p 96 u								500 Met
	12:20 pm	p 94 u								
	5:25 pm	p 80 u								250 Met
	5:25 pm	p E -								Worked Almost All Day Great-Lots of exercise
	10:05 pm	p 97 u								500 Met-Large Pc Apple Pie Last Nit
06/04/06 Sun	7:50 am	p 97 u								Ate Pizza/BR Sticks-@ 9:30 PM
	9:30 pm	p 87 u								500 Met-Pizza/BR Sticks-Bad Boy!
06/05/06 Mon	8:00 am	p 130 u								250 Met-Back on track
	4:40 pm	p 93 u								
	9:50 pm	p 84 u								
06/06/06 Tue	7:00 am	p 96 u								500 Met
	5:00 pm	p 81 u								250 Met
	9:55 pm	p 95 u								
06/07/06 Wed	7:55 am	p 101 u								500 Met
	11:50 am	p 126 u								No explanation--very late breakfast!
	5:15 pm	p 84 u								250 Met
	10:00 pm	p 93 u								great-Lots of exercise today!
06/08/06 Thu	8:00 am	p 104 u								500 Met
	12:05 pm	p 108 u								
	4:50 pm	p 96 u								250 Met
	9:45 pm	p 101 u								

Date	Time	Glucose	Comment
06/09/06 Fri	7:20 am	p 95 u	500 Met
	11:00 am	p 115 u	@ INDY Airport
	3:00 pm	p 92 u	250 Met-On The Way To SF
06/10/06 Sat	9:25 am	p 121 u	500 Met-Late Meds-In CA
	3:00 pm	p 101 u	
	8:00 pm	137 u	250 Met-Late Again/Stress/CA
06/11/06 Sun	9:40 am	p 107 u	500 met
	7:00 pm	p 93 u	250 Met
	11:55 pm	p 96 u	
06/12/06 Mon	10:15 am	p 116 u	500 Met
	3:00 pm	p 93 u	
	9:30 pm	p 90 u	250 Met-Ate Large Meal/While Flour
06/13/06 Tue	11:30 am	p 133 u	500 Met-Stress/While Flour Last Nit
	12:45 pm	157 u	Stress/Meal Times Off/Last Night
	3:00 pm	102 u	250 met
	4:30 pm	p 94 u	
06/14/06 Wed	9:30 am	p 131 u	500 Met
	11:15 am	p 137 u	
	5:00 pm	p 90 u	
06/15/06 Thu	1:15 am	p 89 u	250 Met/Minneapolis
	6:30 am	91 u	Back Home/Mexico/In
	12:25 pm	p 105 u	Normal/500 Met/fast Lab
	5:15 pm	p 98 u	
06/16/06 Fri	7:50 am	p 100 u	250 Met
	12:10 pm	p 104 u	500 Met
	5:10 pm	p 91 uc	No MetFormin!
	9:45 pm	p 80 u	Only 500 Met For The Entire Day!
06/17/06 Sat	7:45 am	p 101 u	500 Met-Great Start-Reducing Breakf
	12:05 pm	p 104 u	
	5:00 pm	p 91 u	0 Metformin!
	10:00 pm	p 88 u	

Date	Time	Glucose	0	40	65	130	180	601	Comment
06/18/06 Sun	8:10 am	p 98 u							500 Met
	1:00 pm	p 103 u							
	10:55 pm	p 110 u							Ate @ 9:00 PM-No Eve Med
06/19/06 Mon	6:45 am	p 91 u							Too Early For Meds *500 Met @ 5:00 pm*
	12:10 pm	p 116 u							
	5:00 pm	p 79 u							No Meds!
	9:00 pm	p 89 u							Berrys/Diet Ice/Nuts
06/20/06 Tue	5:55 am	p 100 u							Too Early For Med
	12:00 pm	p 106 u							
	4:35 pm	p 86 u							
	9:20 pm	p 92 u							
06/21/06 Wed	7:25 am	p 97 u							500 Met
	12:20 pm	p 107 u							
	5:20 pm	p 83 u							
	9:05 pm	p 110 u							Chiken- Sauce @ 9G/Too Large
06/22/06 Thu	8:00 am	p 94 u							500 Met

500 met (handwritten note in graph area)

Date	Time	Glucose		0	40	65	130	180	601	Comment
06/22/06 Thu	8:00 am	p	94 u							500 Met
	12:00 pm	p	116 u							
	5:55 pm	p	94 u							
	9:30 pm	p	93 u							
06/23/06 Fri	7:45 am	p	101 u							500 Met
	12:00 pm	p	100 u							
	5:00 pm	p	97 u							
	9:30 pm	p	90 u							
06/24/06 Sat	7:25 am	p	100 u							Berries-Nuts-Diet Ice Cream/Cho Cks
	5:00 pm	p	115 u							500 Met-Heading To Nashville, IN
	9:55 pm	p	144 u							Diet Ice Cream @ 2:30 PM
										Ate Fried Biscuits for Large dinner
06/25/06 Sun	9:15 am	p	104 u							500 Met
	5:30 pm	p	87 u							Retuned From Nashville, In
	9:05 pm	p	79 u							
06/26/06 Mon	7:20 am	p	92 uc							Breakfast Medicin Reduction 250 Met
	12:10 pm	p	102 u							
	5:00 pm	p	91 u							
	10:45 pm	p	87 u							
06/27/06 Tue	7:20 am	p	88 u							250 Met
	12:00 pm	p	88 u							
	5:00 pm	p	79 u							
	9:10 pm	p	81 u							
06/28/06 Wed	7:00 am	p	99 u							250 Met
	12:10 pm	p	100 u							
	5:00 pm	p	82 u							
	9:05 pm	p	82 u							
06/29/06 Thu	7:05 am	p	85 u							250 Met
	12:10 pm		98 u							
	5:55 pm	p	84 u							
	10:30 pm	p	81 u							
06/30/06 Fri	6:45 am	p	94 u							250 Met-Ron Surgery Today @ 1:00 PM

188

Date	Time	Glucose	0	40	65	130	180	601	Comment
06/30/06 Fri	12:10 pm	p 130 u							Hardees breakfast Sandwiches-2
	4:50 pm	p 83 u							
	9:30 pm	p 95 u							Berries/Nuts/Ice Cream/Choc Chunks
07/01/06 Sat	5:55 am	p 91 u							250 Met
	12:10 pm	p 95 u							
	5:15 pm	p 80 u							
	7:50 pm	85 u							
	9:45 pm	p 93 u							Berries Nuts Ice Cream Choc Chunks
07/02/06 Sun	7:40 am	p 89 u							250 Met
	12:25 pm	p 115 u							
	4:40 pm	p 92 u							
	9:00 pm	p 80 u							
07/03/06 Mon	7:40 am	p 100 u							250 Met
	12:00 pm	p 103 u							
	5:30 pm	p 88 u							
	8:50 pm	p 104 u							
07/04/06 Tue	7:10 am	p 95 u							250 Met
	12:40 pm	p 96 u							
	5:40 pm	p 80 u							Pizza/Bread Sticks & too Much!
	9:30 pm	p 152 u							Watermelon/Nuts-See Dinner
07/05/06 Wed	7:05 am	p 111 u							250 Met-Little Higher Than Norm/Piz
	12:40 pm	p 105 u							
	5:35 pm	p 58 u							Wow!
	9:15 pm	p 88 u							
07/06/06 Thu	7:05 am	p 95 u							250 Met
	12:05 pm	p 100 u							
	5:25 pm	p 84 u							
07/07/06 Fri	7:05 am	p 98 u							250 Met
	12:30 pm	p 109 u							
	5:05 pm	p 80 u							
	9:10 pm	p 96 u							

Date	Time	Glucose	0	40	65	130	180	601	Comment
07/08/06 Sat	7:30 am	p 94 u							250 Met
	12:10 pm	p 107 u							
	5:25 pm	p 82 u							
	9:40 pm	p 110 u							
07/09/06 Sun	7:30 am	p 98 u							250 Met
	11:45 am	p 97 u							
	4:35 pm	p 97 u							
	8:45 pm	p 90 u							
07/10/06 Mon	6:40 am	p 88 u							250 Met
	12:15 pm	p 78 u							
	4:50 pm	p 81 u							
	9:10 pm	p 97 u							
07/11/06 Tue	7:05 am	p 90 u							250 Met
	12:20 pm	p 111 u							
	5:05 pm	p 83 u							
	9:10 pm	p 102 u							
07/12/06 Wed	1:50 am	107 u							Random Check
	7:15 am	p 95 u							250 Met
	12:00 pm	p 100 u							101
	5:30 pm	p 91 u							
	9:20 pm	p 92 u							
07/13/06 Thu	8:00 am	100 u							250 Met
	12:15 pm	p 106 u							
	5:25 pm	p 106 u							
	9:45 pm	p 98 u							
07/14/06 Fri	6:15 am	p 81 u							250 Met
	12:00 pm	p 102 u							
	5:00 pm	p 84 u							
	9:10 pm	p 97 u							
07/15/06 Sat	6:10 am	p 70 uc							Metformin Eliminated Totally! On Target-No Diabetic Medicine!
	1:15 pm	p 106 u							

Date	Time	Glucose	Comment
07/15/06 Sat	5:45 pm	p 96 u	No Diabetic Medicine For Today!
	9:15 pm	p 91 u	No Diabetic Medicine Today!
07/16/06 Sun	1:00 am	p 96 u	Excellent Status After 4th meal
	7:55 am	p 85 u	Great Start!
	12:10 pm	113 u	
	12:50 pm	p 99 u	
	5:00 pm	p 124 u	Hard Workout 40 Min@95 deg
	7:45 pm	68 u	Outdoor work/Cement Blocks
	11:05 pm	92 u	Ate Several Pieces - W Melon @ 8 PM
07/17/06 Mon	1:20 am	98 u	Super
	4:00 am	107 u	
	7:55 am	p 93 u	
	12:05 pm	p 102 u	
	5:10 pm	p 86 u	Super!
	8:25 pm	p 109 u	
	10:05 pm	p 107 u	
07/18/06 Tue	4:20 am	109 u	
	7:25 am	111 u	
	9:20 am	p 115 u	Worked All Night
	11:55 am	124 u	
	12:45 pm	p 121 u	
	3:00 pm	151 uc	Too Hi 250 Met-Stress?/Hrs @ Work
	5:40 pm	p 114 u	
	9:55 pm	p 114 u	
	11:15 pm	p 126 u	
07/19/06 Wed	5:30 am	98 uc	Excellent Start 125 Met
	10:55 am	117 u	
	11:55 am	p 110 u	
	4:25 pm	p 113 u	
	9:35 pm	p 99 u	Super
07/20/06 Thu	6:20 am	101 u	125 Met

Date	Time	Glucose	0	40	65	130	180	601	Comment
07/20/06 Thu	12:00 pm	p 116 u							
	3:15 pm	104 u							
	10:05 pm	p 88 u							
07/21/06 Fri	7:15 am	p 90 u							125 Met
	11:50 am	p 116 u							Last Night's Tenderloin?
	5:10 pm	p 103 u							
	8:30 pm	p 108 u							
07/22/06 Sat	4:45 am	114 u							Elephant Ears!
	7:10 am	p 99 u							125 Metformin
	12:15 pm	p 110 u							
	5:20 pm	p 89 u							
	9:55 pm	p 110 u							
07/23/06 Sun	8:30 am	p 118 u							Late Meds-125 Met
	12:15 pm	p 144 uc							No Breakfast-PA @ MBC-Deacons Mtg
	12:15 pm	p E -							125 Met-Total 250 For The Day
	4:50 pm	p 119 u							Improving - Still High
	10:00 pm	p 97 u							Back On Track
07/24/06 Mon	7:50 am	p 99 u							125 Met
	12:15 pm	p 110 u							
	5:25 pm	p 94 u							
	9:35 pm	p 89 u							
07/25/06 Tue	7:25 am	p 97 u							125 Met
	12:00 pm	p 105 u							
	4:50 pm	106 u							
	9:20 pm	p 99 u							
07/26/06 Wed	6:30 am	p 92 u							125 Met
	12:30 pm	p 106 u							
	5:50 pm	p 95 u							
	9:20 pm	p 105 u							
07/27/06 Thu	2:15 am	99 u							
	5:00 am	67 u							

Date	Time	Glucose	0	40	65	130	180	601	Comment
07/27/06 Thu	7:30 am	p E -							125 Metformin
	12:05 pm	p 117 u							
	5:00 pm	p 106 u							
	9:10 pm	p 103 u							
07/28/06 Fri	8:00 am	p 102 u							125 met
	12:35 pm	p 119 u							
	5:30 pm	p 97 u							
	9:45 pm	p 111 u							
07/29/06 Sat	7:30 am	p 98 u							125 met
	12:15 pm	p 106 u							
	5:05 pm	p 106 u							
	8:00 pm	116 u							
	9:05 pm	p 103 u							
07/30/06 Sun	8:35 am	p 98 u							125 met
	12:10 pm	p 117 u							
	6:30 pm	p 108 u							
	9:00 pm	126 u							
	10:15 pm	p 112 u							
07/31/06 Mon	5:35 am	101 u							125 Met
	12:25 pm	p 115 u							
	4:25 pm	p 117 u							
	10:00 pm	p 103 u							
08/01/06 Tue	6:55 am	p 98 u							125 Met
	12:05 pm	p 109 u							
	9:15 pm	p 107 u							
08/02/06 Wed	6:55 am	p 92 u							125 met
	11:45 am	p 107 u							
	5:10 pm	p 87 u							
	9:15 pm	p 88 u							excellent
08/03/06 Thu	6:09 am	p 84 u							125 Met
	11:45 am	p 104 u							

193

Date	Time	Glucose	0	40	65	130	180	601	Comment
08/03/06 Thu	5:10 pm	p 97 u							
	9:00 pm	p 97 u							125 Met
08/04/06 Fri	7:50 am	p 78 u							
	12:30 pm	p 89 u							
	5:55 pm	p 85 u							
	9:10 pm	p 105 u							125 met
08/05/06 Sat	7:50 am	p 100 u							
	12:15 pm	p 98 u							Watermelon/nuts/muffins
	5:30 pm	p 91 u							125 Met
08/06/06 Sun	8:45 pm	p 85 u							
	8:05 am	p 84 u							
	12:10 pm	p 107 u							
	3:45 pm	p 88 u							
	10:55 pm	p 89 u							125 Met
08/07/06 Mon	8:15 am	p 75 u							
	12:15 pm	p 99 u							
	5:25 pm	p 78 u							
	8:50 pm	p 97 u							125 Met
08/08/06 Tue	7:55 am	p 92 u							
	12:00 pm	p 108 u							
	5:45 pm	p 93 u							
	8:45 pm	p 91 u							125 Met
08/09/06 Wed	7:20 am	p 114 u							
	12:00 pm	p 85 u							
	6:05 pm	p 102 u							
	9:10 pm	p 95 u							125 Met
08/10/06 Thu	7:45 am	p 108 u							
	11:50 am	100 u							
	8:30 pm	p 97 u							
	9:30 pm	p 96 u							125 Met
08/11/06 Fri	7:30 am								

194

Date	Time	Glucose							Comment
			0	40	65	130	180	601	
08/11/06 Fri	12:25 pm	p 116 u							
	4:00 pm	p 92 u							
	11:30 pm	p 83 u							125 Met
08/12/06 Sat	5:40 am	p 103 u							Ate Breakfast @ Lions-Eggs/Pancakes
	8:35 am	E - DS							
	12:30 pm	p 99 u							
	6:00 pm	p 91 u							
	8:30 pm	p 106 u							
	9:50 pm	p 104 u							Lion Ear-1/2 Tenderloin
08/13/06 Sun	8:10 am	p 104 u							125 Met
	12:05 pm	p 122 u							
	5:00 pm	p 88 u							
	9:50 pm	p 106 u							
08/14/06 Mon	7:30 am	p 95 u							125 Met
	11:55 am	p 109 u							
	5:15 pm	p 92 u							
08/15/06 Tue	7:25 am	p 111 u							125 Met
	12:00 pm	102 u							
	5:00 pm	p 90 u							
	9:00 pm	p 94 u							
08/16/06 Wed	7:45 am	p 108 u							125 Met
	12:20 pm	p 109 u							
	5:00 pm	p 83 u							
	10:00 pm	p 95 u							
08/17/06 Thu	7:35 am	p 97 u							125 Met
	12:30 pm	p 104 u							
	5:10 pm	p 88 u							Pizza Br Stks-Fat-White FLour
	10:00 pm	p 165 u							from Pizza/Br Stks/Whit Flour/Fat
08/18/06 Fri	7:25 am	p 124 u							125 Met
	11:50 am	p 114 u							Back to Normal- From Pizza/Br Stk
	5:20 pm	p 83 u							

195

Date	Time	Glucose	0	40	65	130	180	601	Comment
08/18/06 Fri	9:25 pm	p 97 u							Diet ice cream/berries/nuts
08/19/06 Sat	6:40 am	p 107 u							125 Met
	12:25 pm	p 111 u							
	5:40 pm	p 84 u							
	10:05 pm	p 90 u							
08/20/06 Sun	8:25 am	p 108 u							125 Met
	12:25 pm	p 109 u							
	5:10 pm	p 105 u							
	10:40 pm	p 87 u							
08/21/06 Mon	6:50 am	p 103 u							125 met
	1:45 pm	p 95 u							
	5:35 pm	p 91 u							
	9:00 pm	p 90 u							
08/22/06 Tue	7:30 am	p 90 u							125 Met
	12:25 pm	p 111 u							
	5:40 pm	p 85 u							
	9:10 pm	p 96 u							
08/23/06 Wed	8:05 am	p 101 u							125 Met
	12:15 pm	p 107 u							
	5:15 pm	p 106 u							
	9:00 pm	p 80 u							
08/24/06 Thu	7:15 am	p 90 u							125 Met
	12:10 pm	p 88 u							Tomatoes/Lunch
	4:55 pm	p 83 u							Chili Beans-Too Many!
	8:45 pm	p 99 u							
08/25/06 Fri	7:10 am	p 92 u							125 Met
	11:55 am	p 108 u							
	5:15 pm	p 86 u							
	8:45 pm	p 109 u							
08/26/06 Sat	7:30 am	p 91 u							125 Met
	12:10 pm	p 100 u							

Date	Time	Glucose	0	40	65	130	180	601	Comment
08/26/06 Sat	3:45 pm	p 104 u							
	5:10 pm	p 96 u							
	9:10 pm	p 102 u							125 met
08/27/06 Sun	6:30 am	p 102 u							PA-MBC- Worship Leader
	12:15 pm	p 132 u							
	4:45 pm	p 89 u							Watermelon/Nuts
	8:45 pm	p 90 u							125 Met
08/28/06 Mon	8:05 am	p 98 u							
	12:45 pm	p 111 u							
	4:40 pm	p 90 u							
	9:10 pm	p 101 u							
08/29/06 Tue	7:35 am	p 103 u							125 Met
	12:25 pm	p 115 u							
	5:00 pm	p 92 u							
	9:00 pm	p 116 u							Ate Banana W Icecream & Berries
08/30/06 Wed	6:50 am	p 108 u							125 Met
	12:05 pm	p 113 u							
	4:50 pm	p 93 u							
08/31/06 Thu	8:00 am	p 115 u							125 Met
	12:30 pm	p 116 u							
	5:15 pm	p 100 u							
	8:45 pm	p 106 u							
09/01/06 Fri	7:10 am	p 100 u							125 Met
	11:55 am	p 121 u							
	4:50 pm	p 103 u							
	9:10 pm	p 100 u							
09/02/06 Sat	7:00 am	p 108 u							125 met
	12:00 pm	p 116 u							Went To Kirklin/Dan & Patty's
	5:45 pm	p 87 u							
	9:15 pm	p 95 u							
09/03/06 Sun	8:00 am	p 108 u							125 Met

Date	Time	Glucose	0	40	65	130	180	601	Comment
09/03/06 Sun	11:45 am	p 124 u							PA
	5:45 pm	p 106 u							125 Met
09/04/06 Mon	6:55 am	p 98 u							
	12:15 pm	p 116 u							
	5:05 pm	p 104 u							
	9:00 pm	p 101 u							
09/05/06 Tue	7:55 am	p 99 u							125 Met
	12:05 pm	p 112 u							
	4:40 pm	p 103 u							
	9:50 pm	p 99 u							
09/06/06 Wed	8:30 am	p 102 u							125 Met
	12:45 pm	p 111 u							
	5:25 pm	p 91 u							
	9:05 pm	p 95 u							
09/07/06 Thu	7:00 am	p 100 u							125 Met
	12:10 pm	p 112 u							Mary @ Hosp/Abdomen-since 9 4
	5:00 pm	p 100 u							
	10:15 pm	p 90 u							Elephant Ear/Ice Cream
09/08/06 Fri	7:30 am	p 99 u							125 Met
	12:15 pm	p 115 u							
	5:05 pm	p 101 u							
	9:35 pm	p 93 u							
09/09/06 Sat	8:15 am	p 108 u							Elephant Ear/Nuts
	12:15 pm	p 125 u							125 Met
	3:50 pm	p 107 u							Stress/Fam-Reunion Prep-Pics/Sound
	11:25 pm	p 99 u							Family Reunion-Ate Well-3 hrs ago
09/10/06 Sun	8:15 am	p 112 u							125 Met
	12:05 pm	p 158 u							PA & PA Prep/NJ/MBC
	4:50 pm	p 131 u							Ate 3 White Biscuits At Lunch
	9:30 pm	p 100 u							Back To Norm-PA @ Gilead
09/11/06 Mon	7:45 am	p 114 u							125 Met

198

Date	Time	Glucose	0	40 65	130 180	601	Comment
09/11/06 Mon	12:20 pm	p 124 u					Reducing Meal Sizes
	4:05 pm	p 103 u					
	9:35 pm	p 113 u					
09/12/06 Tue	8:00 am	p 101 u					125 Met
	12:55 pm	p 112 u					
	5:00 pm	p 94 u					Exercise-Lots
	9:00 pm	p 95 u					
09/13/06 Wed	6:45 am	p 95 u					125 Met-Meals are smaller!
	12:10 pm	p 75 u					Hard Exercise-Block Laying
	5:35 pm	p 91 u					
09/14/06 Thu	6:20 am	p 90 u					125 Met
	12:00 pm	p 105 u					
	4:50 pm	p 89 u					
	7:55 pm	p 89 u					Mowing-Digging
	9:00 pm	p 88 u					
09/15/06 Fri	7:45 am	p 89 u					125 Met
	12:20 pm	p 107 u					
	5:00 pm	p 103 u					
	8:30 pm	p 88 u					
09/16/06 Sat	6:20 am	p 92 u					125 Met
	12:30 pm	p 95 u					
	6:10 pm	p 77 u					
	9:10 pm	p 107 u					
09/17/06 Sun	7:45 am	p 106 u					125 Met
	12:30 pm	p 130 u					
	5:20 pm	p 88 u					Mike & Donna
	10:55 pm	p 92 u					125 Met 201.8 LBS!
09/18/06 Mon	7:40 am	p 99 u					Stress
	12:15 pm	p 121 u					
	5:30 pm	p 104 u					
	9:15 pm	p 103 u					Practically No Exercise/Day

199

Date	Time	Glucose	0	40	65	130	180	601	Comment
09/19/06 Tue	7:55 am	p 105 u							125 Met
	12:25 pm	p 125 u							
	4:55 pm	p 108 u							
	9:00 pm	p 96 u							
09/20/06 Wed	6:35 am	p 100 u							125 met
	11:36 am	p 124 u							
	5:00 pm	p 94 u							
	9:05 pm	p 101 u							
09/21/06 Thu	8:15 am	p 92 u							125 Met
	12:30 pm	p 103 u							
	4:20 pm	p 107 u							
	8:00 pm	p 95 u							
09/22/06 Fri	7:50 am	p 104 u							125 Met/Ate Late @ 10:00 AM
	12:30 pm	p 108 u							
	5:15 pm	p 96 u							
	9:05 pm	p 104 u							
09/23/06 Sat	6:00 am	p 89 u							125 Met
	12:10 pm	p 103 u							
	4:50 pm	p 111 u							
	10:30 pm	p 117 u							
09/24/06 Sun	8:00 am	p 103 u							Ate Too Much/New Meat/Supper
	12:15 pm	p 127 u							125 Met/Reducing Meal Sizes
	5:00 pm	p 98 u							Worship Leader
	10:55 pm	p 80 u							
09/25/06 Mon	8:05 am	p 92 u							Meal Sizes Reduced-Mike/Donna
	12:40 pm	p 143 u							125 Met
	4:40 pm	p 99 u							New Jerusalem Practice
	8:35 pm	p 87 u							
09/26/06 Tue	7:50 am	p 93 u							125 Met
	1:20 pm	p 114 u							
	4:40 pm	p 96 u							

Date	Time	Glucose	Comment
09/26/06 Tue	8:45 pm	p 96 u	125 met
09/27/06 Wed	7:30 am	p 97 u	
	12:25 pm	p 115 u	
	5:10 pm	p 92 u	
09/28/06 Thu	7:20 am	p 107 u	125 Met
	12:25 pm	p 84 u	
	4:50 pm	p 105 u	
09/29/06 Fri	6:50 am	p 95 u	105 Met
	12:25 pm	p 121 u	Very Late Breakfast-Around 10:00 AM
	5:15 pm	p 96 u	
09/30/06 Sat	7:20 am	p 107 u	125 Met
	2:40 pm	p 102 u	Went Fishing With John / Ate Late Lunch
	8:55 pm	p 81 u	125 Met
10/01/06 Sun	7:30 am	p 106 u	Church/PA
	12:15 pm	p 129 u	Good Recovery
	4:35 pm	p 94 u	PA Gilead-Outing / Mike&Donna
	10:35 pm	p 91 u	Running Long Hours-Nuell-Stephens
10/02/06 Mon	6:45 am	E - ST	125 Met
	6:50 am	p 86 u	MD Egg/Ham/Cheese Biscuit-Warsaw
	8:20 am	p E - DS	NJ Great Rehearsal W Prayer
	12:15 pm	p 133 u	Large Chili Lunch
	4:50 pm	p 110 u	Large Supper-Chili/Beef
	8:55 pm	p 119 u	Too Early For Metformin 125 met
10/03/06 Tue	4:50 am	p 105 u	Working Long Hours
	12:05 pm	p 94 u	
	6:20 pm	p 84 u	
	8:25 pm	p 106 u	2 hrs after dinner
10/04/06 Wed	5:55 am	p 93 u	125 met
	12:05 pm	p 110 u	
	4:30 pm	p 90 u	
10/05/06 Thu	6:00 am	p 97 u	125 Met

Date	Time	Glucose	Comment
10/05/06 Thu	12:00 pm	p 106 u	
	5:45 pm	p 86 u	Large Dinner
	9:05 pm	p 125 u	125 Met
10/06/06 Fri	7:30 am	p 89 u	
	12:10 pm	p 86 u	
	5:00 pm	p 87 u	
10/07/06 Sat	8:20 am	p 106 u	125 Met
	12:50 pm	p 112 u	
	5:00 pm	p 101 u	
10/08/06 Sun	8:00 am	p 104 u	125 Met-Ate Later
	9:50 am	E - DS	Need To Reduce 3rd & 4th Meals
	12:15 pm	p 128 u	AccuCheck-esetimate
	3:50 pm	p 104 u	
	10:55 pm	p 85 u	
10/09/06 Mon	7:30 am	p 118 u	125 Met-No Known cause
	12:25 pm	p 145 u	New Jerusalem Rehearsal
	5:05 pm	p 97 u	
	10:50 pm	p 89 u	Debbie K In Hospital
10/10/06 Tue	7:45 am	p 98 u	125 Met
	12:00 pm	p 109 u	
	5:05 pm	p 97 u	
	8:05 pm	p 94 u	
10/11/06 Wed	8:00 am	p 88 u	125 Met
	11:50 am	p 109 u	
	5:35 pm	p 83 u	
	9:45 pm	p 92 u	
10/12/06 Thu	8:30 am	p 98 u	125 Met
	11:55 am	p 108 u	
	5:15 pm	p 90 u	
	9:00 pm	p 125 u	Unknow
10/13/06 Fri	7:30 am	p 102 u	125 Met

Chart axis values: 0   40   65   130   180   601

Date	Time	Glucose	0	40	65	130	180	601	Comment
10/13/06 Fri	12:00 pm	p 104 u							Pizza/Bread Sticks/Denver
	6:05 pm	p 89 u							
	11:00 pm	p 224 u							125 Met
10/14/06 Sat	7:25 am	p 105 u							
	12:15 pm	p 132 u							
	9:20 pm	p 100 u							
10/15/06 Sun	8:20 am	p 109 u							125 Met
	12:15 pm	p 122 u							
	3:45 pm	p 101 u							
	10:15 pm	p 93 u							
10/16/06 Mon	8:30 am	p 98 u							125 Met
	12:20 pm	p 105 u							
	5:50 pm	p 82 u							
	9:05 pm	p 93 u							
10/17/06 Tue	7:45 am	p 107 u							125 Met
	12:40 pm	p 112 u							
	9:05 pm	p 110 u							
10/18/06 Wed	8:30 am	p 104 u							125 Met
	12:00 pm	p 107 u							
	3:05 pm	p 87 u							
	8:45 pm	p 81 u							
10/19/06 Thu	8:05 am	p 98 u							125 Met
	12:05 pm	p 118 u							Will's/Thad/Recording
	4:15 pm	p 96 u							
	9:00 pm	p 96 u							
10/20/06 Fri	7:10 am	p 100 u							125 Met
	12:05 pm	p 100 u							Mowing
	5:45 pm	p 90 u							Mowing/Siding
	9:10 pm	p 114 u							Late Supper
10/21/06 Sat	8:30 am	p 102 u							125 Met
	12:00 pm	p 111 u							Mowing

203

Date	Time	Glucose	0	40	65	130	180	601	Comment
10/21/06 Sat	5:15 pm	p 101 u							NJ Practice
	9:00 pm	p 94 u							
10/22/06 Sun	8:25 am	p 103 u							125 Met
	12:00 pm	p 134 u							Sunday Worship Leader
	5:10 pm	p 94 u							
	10:20 pm	p 91 u							
10/23/06 Mon	8:40 am	p 104 u							125 Met
	12:30 pm	p 117 u							
	5:45 pm	p 93 u							
	10:00 pm	p 103 u							
10/24/06 Tue	8:40 am	p 109 u							125 Met
	12:15 pm	p 97 u							
	5:55 pm	p 75 u							
	10:10 pm	p 75 u							
10/25/06 Wed	6:30 am	p 92 u							125 Met
	12:00 pm	p 115 u							
	6:15 pm	p 88 u							
	8:30 pm	p 81 u							
10/26/06 Thu	8:30 am	p 106 u							125 Met
	12:30 pm	p 91 u							
	5:15 pm	p 99 u							
	9:05 pm	p 97 u							
10/27/06 Fri	8:05 am	p 105 u							125 Met
	12:00 pm	p 110 u							
	4:39 pm	p 100 u							
10/28/06 Sat	9:00 am	p 102 u							125 Met
	12:15 pm	p 109 u							
	5:00 pm	p 101 u							
10/29/06 Sun	8:00 am	p 103 u							125 Met
	10:15 pm	p 97 u							
10/30/06 Mon	7:20 am	p 106 u							125 Met

204

Date	Time	Glucose	0	40	65	130	180	601	Comment
10/30/06 Mon	2:20 pm	p 100 u							
	6:25 pm	p 89 u							
	9:25 pm	p 128 u							
10/31/06 Tue	7:45 am	p 109 u							125 Met
	12:20 pm	p 108 u							
	4:45 pm	p 93 u							
11/01/06 Wed	7:10 am	p 101 u							125 Met Holloween excessive
	12:40 pm	p 114 u							
	6:05 pm	E - D							Mexican Food/Wh Flour/Too Much
11/02/06 Thu	7:40 am	p 117 u							125 Met-Too Much Dinner 211.8#
	12:05 pm	p 116 u							
	9:05 pm	p 114 u							
11/03/06 Fri	6:00 am	p 105 u							125 met
	11:05 am	p 116 u							
	4:20 pm	p 86 u							
	9:05 pm	p 128 u							
11/04/06 Sat	7:45 am	p 116 u							125 met
	12:20 pm	p 128 u							Siding Building
	5:50 pm	p 82 u							
11/05/06 Sun	8:30 am	p 105 u							125 Met
	4:50 pm	p 93 u							
	9:05 pm	p 94 u							
11/06/06 Mon	8:00 am	p 116 u							125 Met
	1:15 pm	p 108 u							
	5:25 pm	p 98 u							
	9:25 pm	p 79 u							
11/07/06 Tue	8:00 am	p 102 u							125 Met
	12:30 pm	p 105 u							
	5:05 pm	p 83 u							
	8:15 pm	p 94 u							
11/08/06 Wed	8:00 am	p 112 u							125 Met

Date	Time	Glucose	Comment
11/08/06 Wed	5:00 pm	p 91 u	
	8:05 pm	p 93 u	125 Met-Keep focus on Small Meals
11/09/06 Thu	8:00 am	p 102 u	
	11:15 am	p 96 u	Panel Painting
	4:35 pm	p 86 u	
	9:05 pm	p 94 u	
11/10/06 Fri	8:00 am	p 103 u	125 Met
	12:05 pm	p 103 u	
	5:15 pm	p 84 u	
	9:00 pm	p 103 u	
11/11/06 Sat	8:30 am	p 113 u	125 Met
	12:05 pm	p 122 u	Virus/Cold
	5:30 pm	p 86 u	
11/12/06 Sun	8:30 am	p 105 u	125 Met
	4:45 pm	p 104 u	
	10:15 pm	p 84 u	
11/13/06 Mon	8:25 am	p 99 u	125 Met
	12:00 pm	p 105 u	
	4:40 pm	p 101 u	
	9:25 pm	p 84 u	
11/14/06 Tue	8:10 am	p 99 u	125 Met
	12:15 pm	p 107 u	Exercise Up
	4:30 pm	p 81 u	
	8:40 pm	p 89 u	
11/15/06 Wed	7:45 am	p 100 u	125 Met
	12:15 pm	p 97 u	Kepp Focus/Small Meals
	5:05 pm	p 81 u	
	9:00 pm	p 96 u	
11/16/06 Thu	8:10 am	p 91 u	125 Met
	12:30 pm	p 96 u	Looking Much Better
	5:00 pm	p 86 u	

Date	Time	Glucose	Comment
5/06 Thu	9:00 pm	p 98 u	125 Met
7/06 Fri	8:20 am	p 94 u	
	12:05 pm	p 104 u	
	9:05 pm	p 101 u	First Eye Medication-Travoprost
8/06 Sat	11:30 pm	E - S	
	7:55 am	p 94 u	125 Met
	12:40 pm	p 103 u	
	5:15 pm	p 74 u	
	9:10 pm	p 92 u	
9/06 Sun	8:25 am	p 98 u	125 Met
	12:10 pm	p 101 u	
	4:35 pm	p 89 u	
	10:20 pm	p 93 u	
0/06 Mon	7:50 am	p 95 u	125 Met / NJ Rehearsal
	12:20 pm	p 112 u	
	5:40 pm	p 88 u	
	9:25 pm	p 97 u	Added Nutbread to last meal
1/06 Tue	8:00 am	p 97 u	125 Met
	12:10 pm	p 112 u	
	5:20 pm	p 89 u	
	8:30 pm	p 105 u	
2/06 Wed	8:30 am	p 98 u	125 Met-Curb Liquids
	12:05 pm	p 97 u	
	5:20 pm	p 90 u	
	9:05 pm	p 107 u	
3/06 Thu	8:00 am	p 104 u	125 Met-Weight 212.4-too high!
	12:10 pm	p 113 u	
	5:35 pm	p 90 u	
	9:00 pm	p 106 u	Ice Cream W/O Berries
4/06 Fri	8:30 am	p 82 u	125 Met-No Berries Last Night
	12:45 pm	p 98 u	

Chart scale: 0   40   65   130   180   601

Date	Time	Glucose	0	40 65	130	180	601	Comment
11/24/06 Fri	5:15 pm	p 79 u						Super Day/NJ Rehearsal
	8:20 pm	p 98 u						125 Met
11/25/06 Sat	7:45 am	p 100 u						
	12:20 pm	p 113 u						
	5:45 pm	p 88 u						
	8:10 pm	p 84 u						Two pieces Of Pie Now
11/26/06 Sun	7:55 am	p 108 u						125 Met
	12:10 pm	p 127 u						Worship Leader
	4:15 pm	p 104 u						
	10:40 pm	p 105 u						
11/27/06 Mon	8:10 am	p 126 u						NJ @ Gilead
	1:10 pm	p 132 u						125 Met
	6:00 pm	p 96 u						NJ Rehearsal
	9:05 pm	p 91 u						
11/28/06 Tue	8:05 am	p 99 u						125 Met
	12:15 pm	p 130 u						
	5:25 pm	p 97 u						
	9:25 pm	p 116 u						
11/29/06 Wed	8:15 am	p 103 u						125 Met
	1:05 pm	p 113 u						
	7:00 pm	p 89 u						
	9:35 pm	p 80 u						
11/30/06 Thu	8:40 am	p 87 u						125 Met
	12:15 pm	p 98 u						
	4:45 pm	E - ST						Injured Back/Cast Iron Tub Move
	4:55 pm	p 91 u						
	7:50 pm	p 90 u						
12/01/06 Fri	8:20 am	p 95 u						125 Met
	11:50 pm	p 105 u						
	4:50 pm	p 92 u						
	8:00 pm	p 82 u						

Date	Time	Glucose	0	40	65	130	180	601	Comment
12/02/06 Sat	7:30 am	p 96 u							125 Met
	12:00 pm	p 102 u							
	4:00 pm	p 116 u							PA Jackson St Peru Baptist
	8:00 pm	p 110 u							PA @ Fundraiser
12/03/06 Sun	8:00 am	p 102 u							125 Met
	12:00 pm	p 112 u							
	4:50 pm	p 95 u							
	10:00 pm	p 92 u							
12/04/06 Mon	7:45 am	p 96 u							
	12:00 pm	114 u							REHEARSAL
	5:00 pm	101 u P							read 30 min After eating
	9:10 pm	p 106 u							
12/05/06 Tue	8:05 am	p 86 u							125 Met
	12:00 pm	p 104 u							
	5:00 pm	p 78 u							Migrane @ 2:30 PM
	8:50 pm	p 104 u							
12/06/06 Wed	7:35 am	p 97 u							125 Met
	12:00 pm	p 102 u							
	5:00 pm	p 88 u							
	9:00 pm	p 102 u							
12/07/06 Thu	7:35 am	p 100 u							125 Met
	11:50 am	p 115 u							
	5:50 pm	p 89 u							
	8:20 pm	p 109 u							Only 2 1/2 Hrs-
12/08/06 Fri	7:00 am	p 100 u							125 Met
	9:14 am	E - S							PrepareTo Reduce Reading Frequency
	12:05 pm	p 103 u							
	5:00 pm	p 105 u							
	9:05 pm	p 83 u							
12/09/06 Sat	8:20 am	p 106 u							125 Met
	5:00 pm	p 93 u							|"

Date	Time	Glucose	0	40	65	130	180	601	Comment
12/09/06 Sat	8:40 pm	p 103 u							125 Met
12/10/06 Sun	8:10 am	p 113 u							NJ Rehearsal
	12:05 pm	p 132 u							
	4:30 pm	p 100 u							
	8:30 pm	p 97 u							
12/11/06 Mon	8:10 am	p 101 u							125 Met
	12:20 pm	p 118 u							
	5:00 pm	p 93 u							
	9:30 pm	p 110 u							
12/12/06 Tue	1:50 am	p 128 u							125 Met
	9:20 am	p 117 u							
	12:10 pm	p 123 u							
	8:55 pm	p 95 u							
12/13/06 Wed	8:00 am	p 112 u							125 Met
	11:50 am	p 125 u							
	4:45 pm	p 95 u							
	9:20 pm	p 107 u							
12/14/06 Thu	8:00 am	p 111 u							125 Met
	1:00 pm	p 112 u							
	6:50 pm	p 97 u							About 2 1/2 hrs Betwee meals
	9:25 pm	p 124 u							125 Met Forgot Breakfast
12/15/06 Fri	8:30 am	p 107 u							Forgot Breakfast
	12:15 pm	p 120 u							
	4:30 pm	p 105 u							
12/16/06 Sat	8:35 am	p 109 u							125 Met
	12:25 pm	p 118 u							
	5:45 pm	p 91 u							
	9:15 pm	p 112 u							
12/17/06 Sun	8:30 am	p 106 u							125 Met
	12:15 pm	p 132 u							
	4:30 pm	p 98 u							

Date	Time	Glucose	0	40	65	130	180	601	Comment
12/17/06 Sun	10:25 pm	p 94 u							125 Met
12/18/06 Mon	8:10 am	p 115 u							
	12:15 pm	p 130 u							
	4:40 pm	p 106 u							
	9:00 pm	p 98 u							
12/19/06 Tue	7:15 am	p 110 u							125 Met
	11:45 am	p 115 u							
	4:45 pm	p 102 u							
12/20/06 Wed	4:45 pm	p 113 u							125 Met-Debbie To Surgery
	6:00 pm	p 94 u							
	9:30 pm	p 132 u							
12/21/06 Thu	8:05 am	p 119 u							125 Met
	12:00 pm	p 126 u							
	5:00 pm	p 107 u							
	10:00 pm	p 103 u							
12/22/06 Fri	7:50 am	p 116 u							125 Met
	12:55 pm	p 121 u							
	4:40 pm	p 131 u							
	9:30 pm	p 131 u							Have A Cold-Weight is @ 212
12/23/06 Sat	6:50 am	p 111 u							125 Met
	12:30 pm	p 112 u							
	6:00 pm	p 110 u							Weight @ 214.4
	9:30 pm	p 133 u							Have A Bad Cold-Weigh Too Much
12/24/06 Sun	6:30 am	p 110 u							125 Met Weight @ 216.4
12/25/06 Mon	9:50 am	p 117 u							125 Met Weight @ 216.4
	2:00 pm	p 109 u							Weight @ 216.4
	6:10 pm	p 120 u							Bad Cold/Virus
12/26/06 Tue	8:20 am	p 113 u							175 Met Weight @ 216.6
	12:15 pm	p 112 u							
	1:20 pm	E - DISTY P							Migraine/Travatan?/Ibuprofin?
	7:30 pm	p 133 u							Bad Cold/Post Migraine

Date	Time	Glucose	Comment
12/27/06 Wed	8:05 am	p 117 u	175 Met Cold Improving Wt @ 213.6
	11:30 am	p 128 u	Cold Improving
	4:10 pm	p 110 u	Cold Improving
	8:50 pm	p 90 u	Finally Back To Normal
12/28/06 Thu	7:55 am	p 110 u	175 Met -- Weight @ 212.6
	11:50 am	p 116 u	
	5:00 pm	p 97 u	Improving
	9:00 pm	p 128 u	
12/29/06 Fri	7:55 am	p 110 u	175 Met Weight @ 213.2
	12:15 pm	p 112 u	
	5:00 pm	p 92 u	
	9:00 pm	p 96 u	
12/30/06 Sat	7:15 am	p 99 u	125 Met
	9:50 pm	p 79 u	Cold Abating
12/31/06 Sun	8:05 am	p 102 u	150 Met
	11:40 am	p 113 u	
	3:45 pm	p 103 u	Early Lunch
	10:00 pm	p 108 u	
01/01/07 Mon	10:00 am	p 109 u	175 Met
01/02/07 Tue	8:00 am	p 121 u	125 Met
	12:10 pm	p 119 u	
	6:35 pm	p 86 u	
	9:30 pm	p 103 u	Cold Abating
01/03/07 Wed	8:45 am	p 119 u	125 Met
	12:30 pm	p 114 u	
	5:15 pm	p 88 u	
	9:45 pm	p 98 u	
01/04/07 Thu	8:20 am	p 107 u	Cold Abating
	12:10 pm	p 108 u	125 Met
	4:25 pm	p 86 u	
	8:15 pm	p 111 u	

Chart axis labels: 0   40   65   130   180   601

Date	Time	Glucose	0	40 65	130	180	601	Comment
01/05/07 Fri	8:15 am	p 116 u						125 Met
	12:40 pm	p 119 u						
	5:10 pm	p 94 u						
	9:10 pm	p 111 u						
01/06/07 Sat	8:05 am	p 109 u						125 Met
	12:20 pm	p 108 u						
	4:50 pm	p 102 u						
	9:45 pm	p 101 u						
01/07/07 Sun	3:30 am	p 117 u						Random Early Morn check .. 30 Met
	8:30 am	p 115 u						125 Met
	8:30 am	E - S						Focus On Smaller Meal Sizes
	4:25 pm	p 90 u						
	10:05 pm	p 119 u						Public Appearance/Gilead Singers
01/08/07 Mon	8:20 am	p 111 u						175 Met
	12:05 pm	p 72 u						Exercise
	5:00 pm	p 94 u						
	8:45 pm	p 105 u						
01/09/07 Tue	8:10 am	p 106 u						
	12:00 pm	p 109 u						175 met
	5:00 pm	p 94 u						
	9:40 pm	p 106 u						
01/10/07 Wed	8:20 am	p 100 u						175 Met
	12:40 pm	p 115 u						
	5:20 pm	p 91 u						
	8:30 pm	p 104 u						
01/11/07 Thu	8:05 am	p 109 u						200 Met
	12:10 pm	p 123 u						Unknown Cause
	4:20 pm	p 96 u						
	9:35 pm	p 89 u						
01/12/07 Fri	7:00 am	p 105 u						125 Met
	12:10 pm	p 99 u						

213

Date	Time	Glucose		0	40	65	130	180	601	Comment
01/12/07 Fri	3:30 pm	E - ST								Tim & Sue Getting Divorce ate @ 5:30 PM
	4:20 pm	p 103 u								
	9:00 pm	p 93 u								
01/13/07 Sat	8:20 am	p 105 u								175 Met
	12:25 pm	p 107 u								Improving Computer Entry Frequency
	5:20 pm	p 99 u								
01/14/07 Sun	8:40 am	p 130 u								175 Met Ate White Flour Last Night
	4:30 pm	p 99 u								Back On Track
	9:55 pm	p 104 u								Could not meet with Mike & Donna
01/15/07 Mon	6:00 am	p 96 u								175 Met
	12:20 pm	p 107 u								
	5:10 pm	p 107 u								
01/16/07 Tue	8:25 pm	p 95 u								
	7:15 am	p 100 u								
	12:05 pm	p 114 u								
	5:10 pm	p 104 u								
	9:20 pm	p 89 u								
01/17/07 Wed	8:05 am	p 109 u								175 Met
	12:30 pm	p 128 u								
	6:30 pm	p 107 u								
	10:05 pm	105 u								
01/18/07 Thu	8:35 am	p 115 u								175 Met
	12:20 pm	p 108 u								
	5:00 pm	p 90 u								
01/19/07 Fri	8:30 pm	p 154 u								Tim & Sue's troubles
	8:10 am	p 120 u								175 Met/Weigh too much
	12:10 pm	p 120 u								
	5:00 pm	p 110 u								
01/20/07 Sat	9:20 pm	p 130 u								Stress-Mindy Has Cancer
	8:25 am	p 120 u								175 Met
	12:25 pm	p 118 u								Stress

214

Date	Time	Glucose	0	40	65	130	180	601	Comment
01/20/07 Sat	6:10 pm	p 100 u							Stress
	9:30 pm	p 122 u							175 Met
01/21/07 Sun	8:30 am	p 113 u							Worship Leader
	12:00 pm	p 143 u							
	4:30 pm	p 109 u							
	8:40 pm	p 102 u							Missed Donna & Mike Tonight
01/22/07 Mon	8:35 am	p 105 u							175 Met/Better Daily Start
	12:15 pm	p 123 u							
	5:25 pm	p 95 u							Better
	9:15 pm	p 120 u							Too High-Still Weigh too much
01/23/07 Tue	8:35 am	p 116 u							175 Met
	11:30 am	p 123 u							
	5:00 pm	p 86 u							Dukes Hospital/Debbie K
	9:00 pm	p 110 u							Still Too High
01/24/07 Wed	8:00 am	p 113 u							175 Met
	12:10 pm	p 120 u							
	4:30 pm	p 107 u							
	7:45 pm	p 88 u							
01/25/07 Thu	8:00 am	p 107 u							175 Met
	12:20 pm	p 113 u							
	5:05 pm	p 93 u							
	9:00 pm	p 112 u							
01/26/07 Fri	8:20 am	p 120 u							175 Met
	11:20 am	p 119 u							Mindy To Surgery @ 2:00 PM
	5:30 pm	p 90 u							Mindy Out Of Surgery-
	10:30 pm	p 86 u							Mindy Released
01/27/07 Sat	8:10 am	p 130 u							175 Met
	12:30 pm	p 128 u							Stress
	4:25 pm	p 109 u							Stress
	9:05 pm	p 106 u							
01/28/07 Sun	7:45 am	p 112 u							175 Met

Date	Time	Glucose	0	40	65	130	180	601	Comment
01/28/07 Sun	12:10 pm	p 140 u				■			Worship Leader-Jim Resigned-Stress
	4:40 pm	p 122 u				■			
	10:15 pm	p 102 u			■				
01/29/07 Mon	6:00 am	p 112 u			■				175 met
	12:05 pm	p 133 u				■			
	4:50 pm	p 99 u			■				
	9:00 pm	p 94 u			■				
01/30/07 Tue	8:30 am	p 125 u				■			
	12:15 pm	p 133 u				■			
	4:30 pm	p 102 u			■				
	10:40 pm	p 102 u			■				
01/31/07 Wed	8:30 am	p 126 u				■			
	12:45 pm	p 127 u				■			
	12:45 pm	E - S							Comp Entry Failure 1 30 07-2 14 07
	4:00 pm	p 73 u		■					
02/01/07 Thu	9:00 am	p 139 u				■			
	12:20 pm	p 145 u				■			
	5:15 pm	p 89 u			■				
	8:35 pm	p 102 u			■				
02/02/07 Fri	8:10 am	p 119 u				■			
	12:45 pm	p 121 u				■			
	2:00 pm	E - ST							Rachel Has Surgery/Galbladder
	4:20 pm	p 107 u			■				
02/03/07 Sat	8:50 am	p 119 u				■			
	12:30 pm	p 136 u				■			
	1:55 pm	p 125 u				■			
	5:25 pm	p 92 u			■				
02/04/07 Sun	8:15 am	p 117 u			■				
	12:15 pm	p 154 u				■			Worship Leader/Stress
	4:30 pm	p 94 u			■				
	11:00 pm	p 98 u			■				SuperBowl Sunday

Date	Time	Glucose	0	40	65	130	180	601	Comment
02/05/07 Mon	8:00 am	p 110 u							Toni Has Cancer/Ovarian
	12:00 pm	p 115 u							
	2:00 pm	E - ST							
	4:10 pm	p 110 u							
	11:30 pm	p 111 u							
02/06/07 Tue	8:00 am	p 108 u							
	12:00 pm	p 111 u							
	5:00 pm	p 104 u							
	9:10 pm	p 119 u							
02/07/07 Wed	8:00 am	p 104 u							
	12:00 pm	p 126 u							
	4:20 pm	p 113 u							
	9:00 pm	p 108 u							
02/08/07 Thu	9:00 am	p 116 u							
	12:00 pm	p 113 u							
	5:20 pm	p 96 u							
	9:20 pm	p 95 u							
02/09/07 Fri	8:00 am	p 120 u							
	12:25 pm	p 118 u							
	5:15 pm	p 96 u							
	9:20 pm	p 113 u							
02/10/07 Sat	8:55 am	p 109 u							
	12:00 pm	p 130 u							
	4:30 pm	p 97 u							
	9:30 pm	p 109 u							
02/11/07 Sun	8:25 am	p 113 u							Sunday Worship
	12:00 pm	p 159 u							
	5:15 pm	p 112 u							
	11:30 pm	p 111 u							
02/12/07 Mon	5:15 am	p 148 u							Stress & Weight
	11:30 am	p 125 u							

Date	Time	Glucose	0	40	65	130	180	601	Comment
02/12/07 Mon	5:00 pm	p 101 u							
	8:05 pm	p 100 u							
02/13/07 Tue	12:15 pm	p 126 u							Exercise-Snow shoveling
	5:30 pm	p 105 u							
	9:00 pm	p 90 u							
02/14/07 Wed	8:20 am	p 120 u							
	11:50 am	p 117 u							Exercise-Snow Shoveling
	4:25 pm	p 87 u							

218

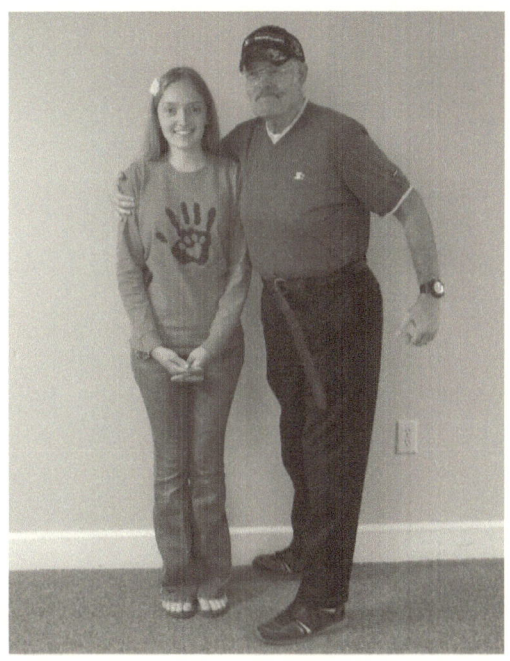

In closing, we just want to say "Remember to stay humble, anticipate success, read, record (document), and analyze the information about yourself, for which you have invested time."

Make certain to Pray daily and give GOD the credit for your success.

And, in the midst of all of this, may HOPE be your constant companion!

www.ingramcontent.com/pod-product-compliance
Lightning Source LLC
Chambersburg PA
CBHW030429290526
45786CB00001B/212